Gynaecological Malignancies - Updates and Advances

Edited by Gwo Yaw Ho and Sophia Frentzas

Published in London, United Kingdom

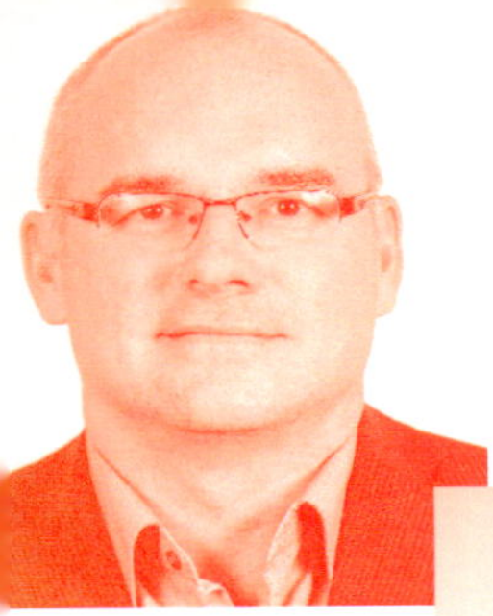
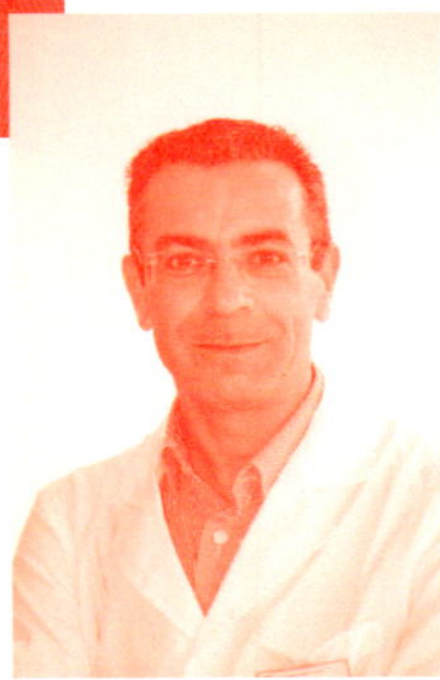
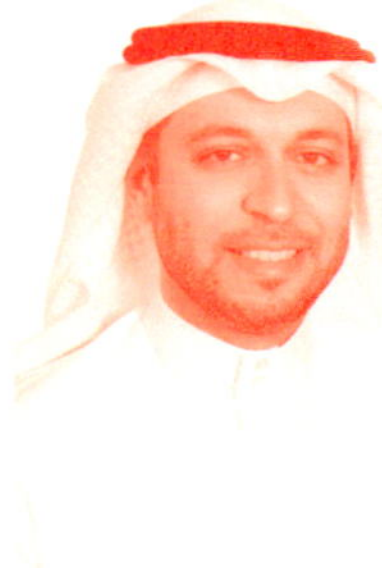
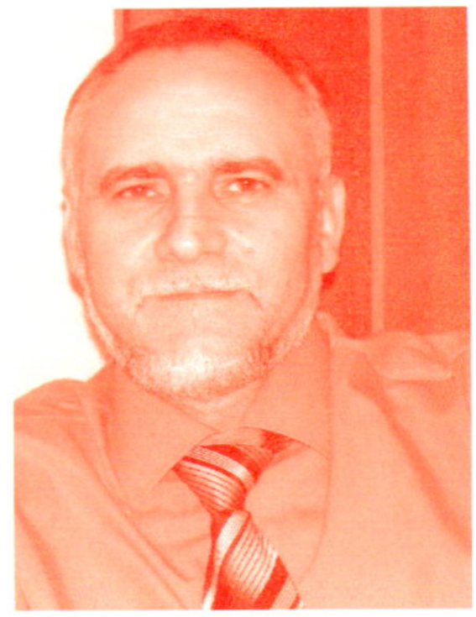
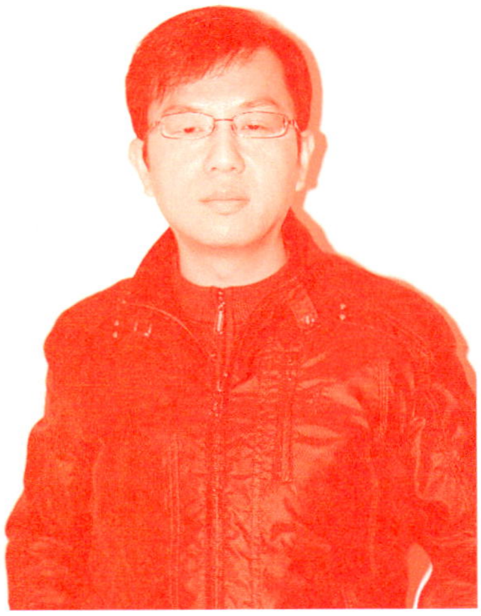
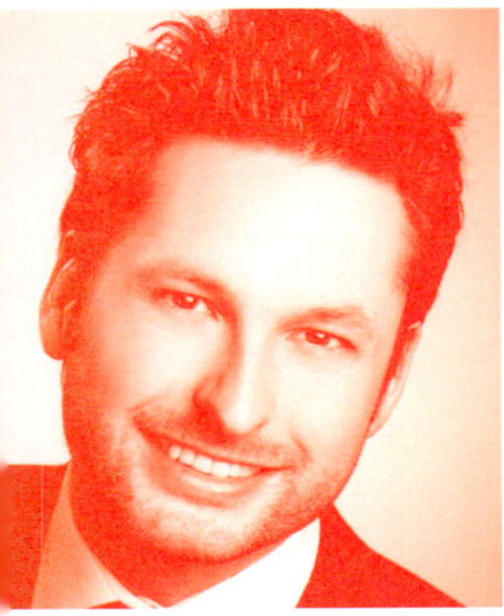
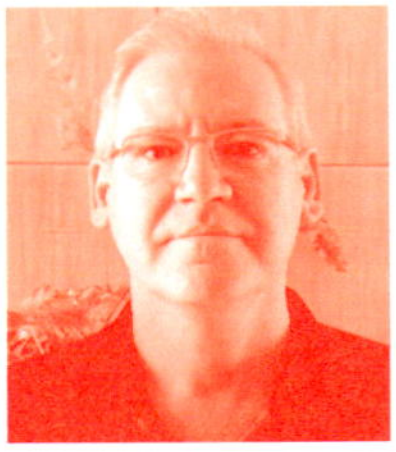

IntechOpen

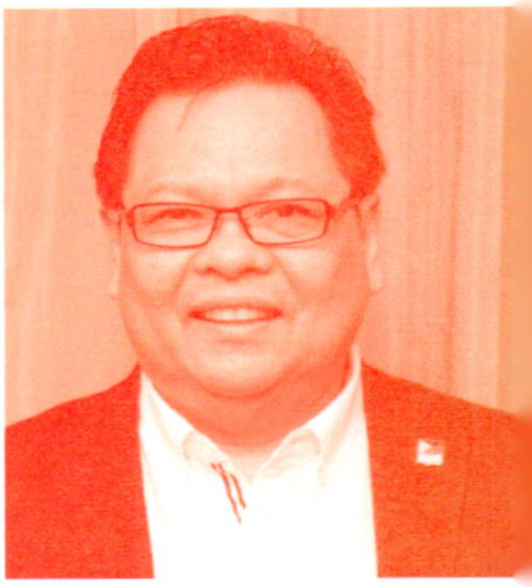
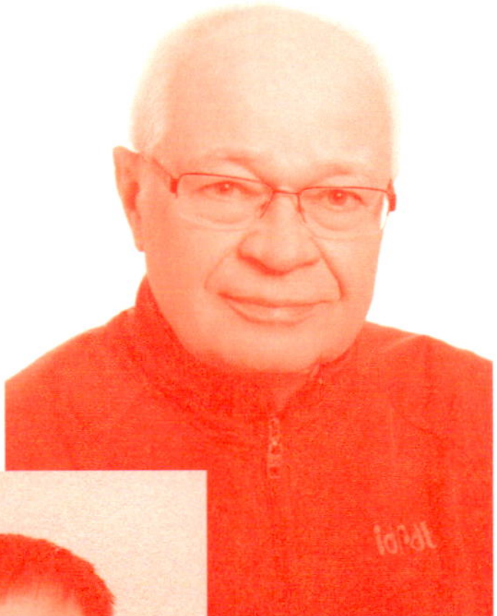
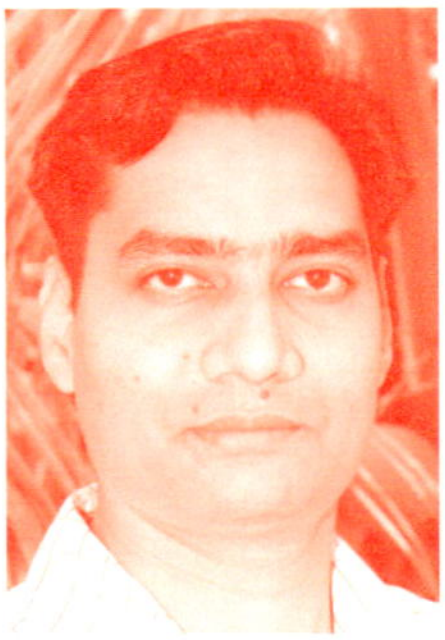
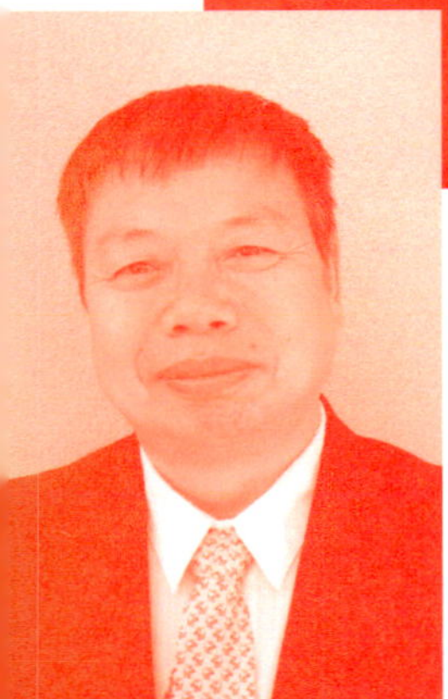
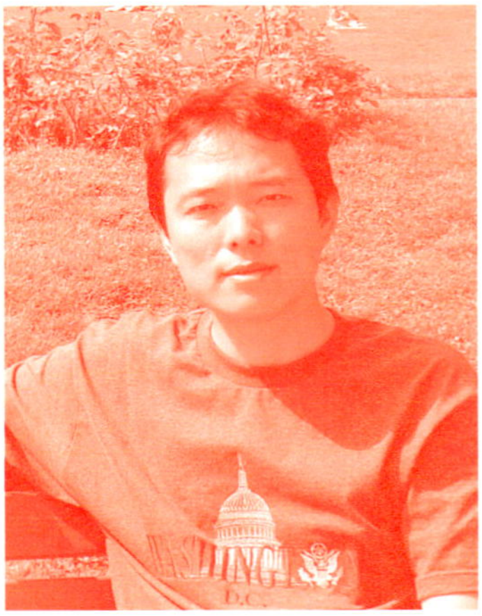
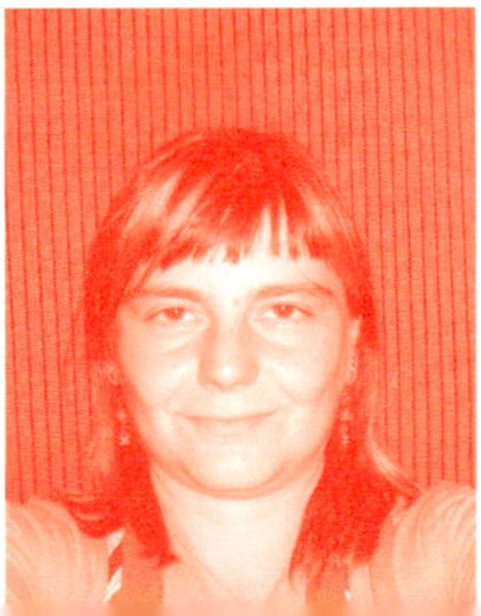

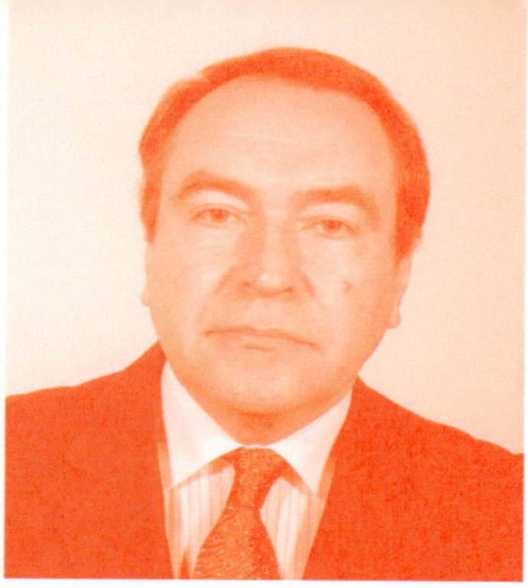
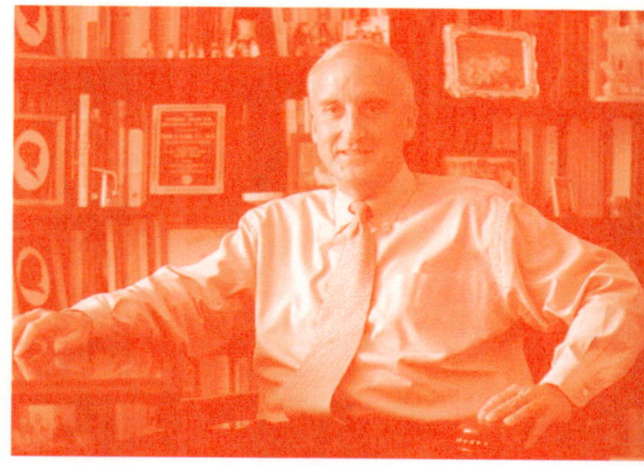
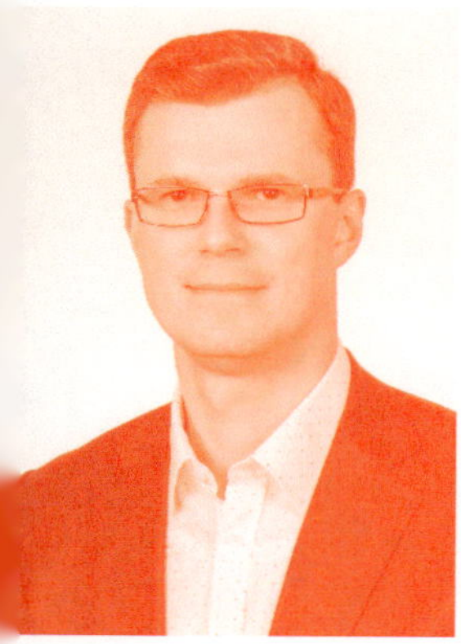
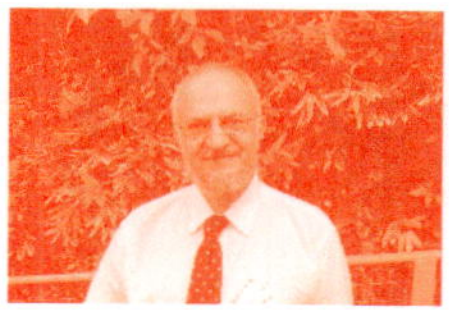
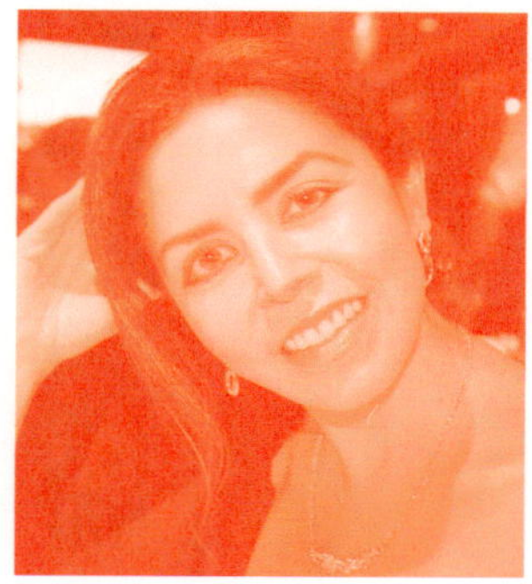

Supporting open minds since 2005

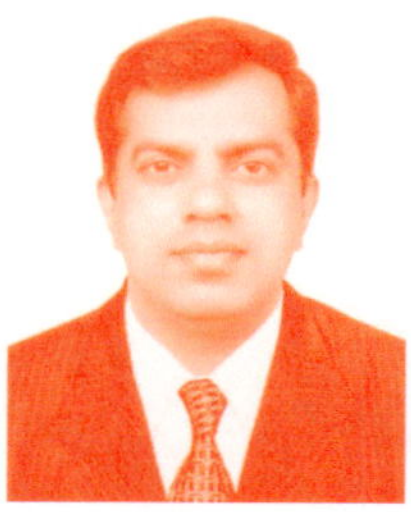
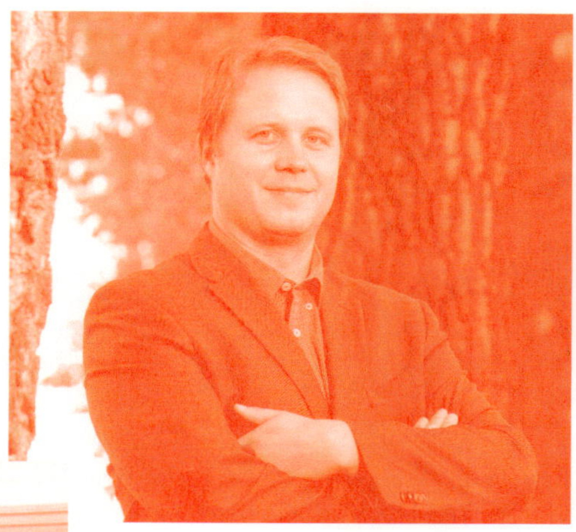
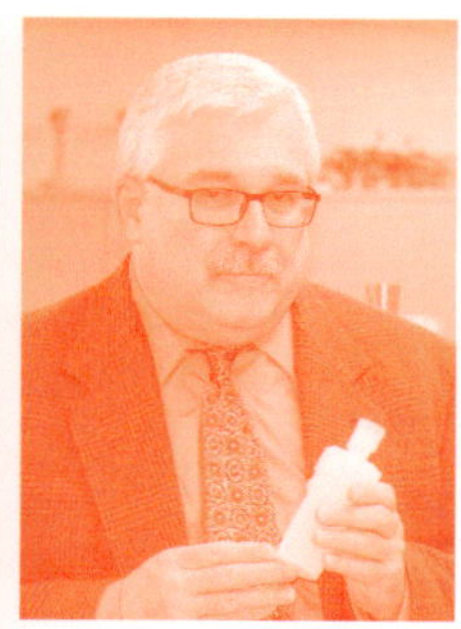
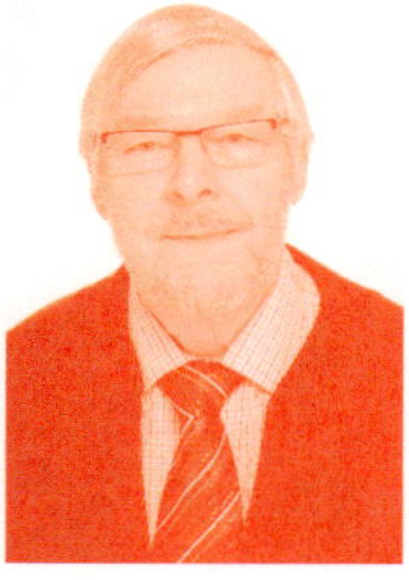
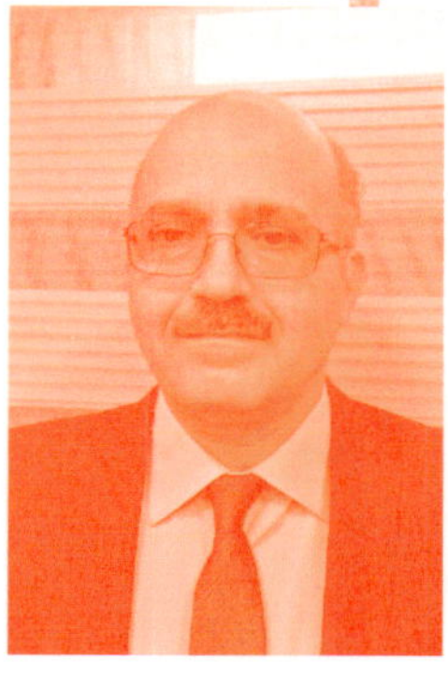
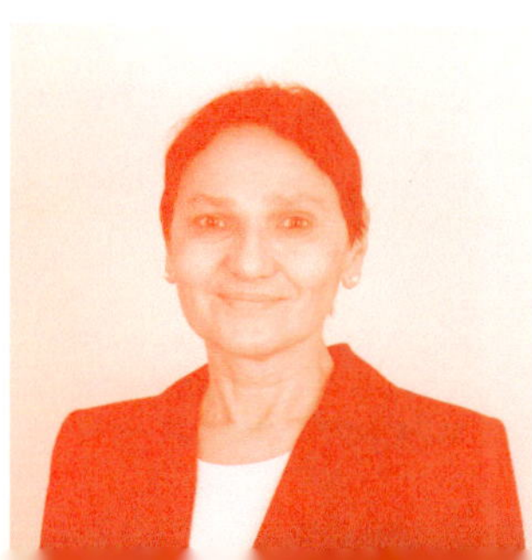
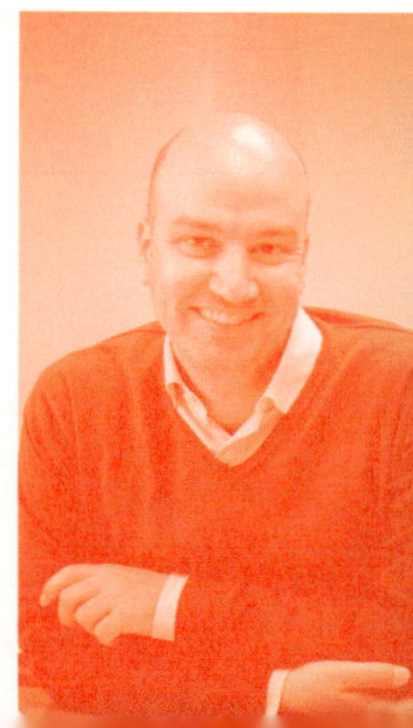

Gynaecological Malignancies - Updates and Advances
http://dx.doi.org/10.5772/intechopen.83164
Edited by Gwo Yaw Ho and Sophia Frentzas

Contributors
Deepti Sharma, Neha Sharma, José Díaz-Chávez, Yair Alfaro-Mora, Marco A. Andonegui-Elguera, Guadalupe Domínguez-Gómez, Luis A Herrera, Rodrigo Cáceres-Gutiérrez, Mai Hazekawa, Takuya Nishinakagawa, Tomoyo Kawakubo-Yasukochi, Manabu Nakashima, Evgeniia Sergeevna Sukhikh, Leonid Grigorievich Sukhikh, Albert Biete, Angeles Rovirosa, Gabriela Oses, Gwo Yaw Ho, Sumitra Ananda, Cassandra J. Vandenberg, Orla McNally, Jeanne Tie, Kylie Gorringe, David Bowtell, Jan Pyman, Matthew J. Wakefield, Clare L. Scott

First published in London, United Kingdom, 2020 by IntechOpen
IntechOpen is the global imprint of INTECHOPEN LIMITED, registered in England and Wales, registration number: 11086078, 7th floor, 10 Lower Thames Street, London, EC3R 6AF, United Kingdom
Printed in Croatia

British Library Cataloguing-in-Publication Data
A catalogue record for this book is available from the British Library

Additional hard and PDF copies can be obtained from orders@intechopen.com

Gynaecological Malignancies - Updates and Advances
Edited by Gwo Yaw Ho and Sophia Frentzas
p. cm.
Print ISBN 978-1-83880-305-6
Online ISBN 978-1-83880-306-3
eBook (PDF) ISBN 978-1-83880-279-0

For EU product safety concerns:
IN TECH d.o.o., Prolaz Marije Krucifikse Kozulić 3, 51000 Rijeka, Croatia, info@intechopen.com or visit our website at intechopen.com.

Meet the editorS

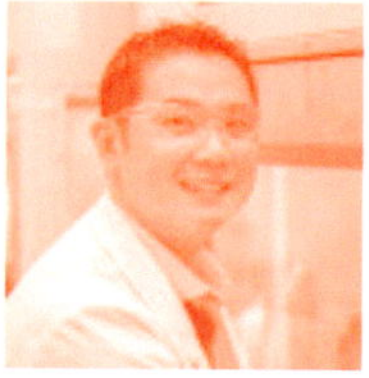

Gwo Yaw Ho is a senior medical oncologist at Monash Health and he specialises in treating women with breast and gynaecologic cancer. He has an academic appointment with Monash University as a research fellow and was awarded the Monash University, School of Clinical Science Clinician-scientist Fellowship in 2019. He completed his PhD study in 2019 at the Walter and Eliza Hall (WEHI) Institute of Medical Research whilst practicing as a medical oncologist at the Peter MacCallum Cancer Centre and Royal Women's Hospital, Melbourne. The focus of his research is a subset of high-grade ovarian cancer, including carcinosarcoma, with the poorest outcome which is associated with increased activity of the oncogenic MYCN pathway.

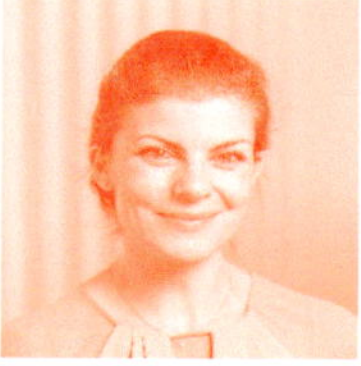

Dr Sophia Frentzas is a medical oncologist and clinical researcher focusing on gynaecological and gastrointestinal malignancies as well as Phase I clinical trials. Dr Frentzas graduated from Imperial College School of Medicine, London, in 2002. She has also completed a laboratory-based, translational PhD at the Institute of Cancer Research, University of London and was awarded her doctorate certificate in 2014. Since migrating to Australia in 2016, Dr Frentzas has worked as a Full Time Specialist in Medical Oncology at the Alan Walker Cancer Centre, Royal Darwin Hospital, NT. During this time, she chaired the Clinical Trials Unit at the Alan Walker Cancer Centre, was a member of the NT Cancer Care Network, was involved in outreach oncology clinic support in the Northern Territory, conducted the Cultural Awareness and Safety course, and participated in The Flinders University medical student teaching program. Dr Frentzas is now part of the medical oncology team at Monash Health where she specialises in the treatment of patients with colorectal, upper gastrointestinal tract, and gynaecological tract cancers. Her main research interests are focused on novel and personal approaches for the treatment of solid tumours, particularly in targeting aberrant pathways for angiogenesis, and on the investigation of strategies to overcome resistance to conventionally employed therapeutic agents. Her research has been published in a number of peer-reviewed, high impact factor journals, and abstracts. She has also had the opportunity to present her work at several national and international conferences.

Contents

Preface

Gynaecological malignancies are a heterogeneous group of diseases composed of multiple types of cancer based on their organ-of-origin within the female genital tract; each type having their own distinct molecular and clinical sub-categorisation. Women with advanced gynaecological malignancy, in particular the rarer subtypes, face a formidable challenge as fatal resistance to therapies commonly occurs within a few years of diagnosis. The improvement in our ability to understand the tumour biology and to target the underlying drivers and vulnerabilities of these tumours is essential in order to develop effective treatments for women battling this disease.

This book aims to present a review of the significant advances in the understanding and management of gynaecological malignancies. Major areas of importance in this field will be covered, incorporating new knowledge that has arisen due to the advancements in molecular techniques and the ability to correlate these molecular changes with clinical behaviour of gynaecologic tumours. The therapeutic implications of molecular subtyping to match appropriate therapies and the appreciation of the use of up-to-date radiotherapy techniques will be explored.

Gwo Yaw Ho
Monash University,
Australia

Walter and Eliza Hall Institute,
Parkville, Australia

Peter MacCallum Cancer Centre,
Melbourne, Australia

Sophia Frentzas
Monash University,
Australia

Section 1

Advances in Gynaecological Malignancies

Chapter 1

Immunotherapy in Gynecological Malignancies

Neha Sharma and Deepti Sharma

Abstract

Cancer immunotherapy is one of the most upcoming treatment strategies emerging as a fascinating option in the management of advanced gynecological malignancies. The development of immune-based antitumor approaches has led to safer treatment options that give fruitful results in these malignancies. In this chapter we are focusing on immune-based treatment in the management of gynecological cancers like cervical cancer, endometrial cancer, ovarian cancer, and vaginal and vulvar cancer. We are also discussing the clinical studies that have been conducted or are currently underway which are exploring these immune strategies that are developing as a logical overture for the treatment of advanced cancers including gynecological cancers.

Keywords: gynecological malignancy, immunotherapy, immune checkpoint inhibitors, cervical cancer, ovarian cancer, endometrial cancer

1. Introduction

Cancer immunotherapy is emerging as an attractive strategy among different therapeutic options over the past years, and also the treatment of many advanced malignancies has been revolutionized with the development of immune-based antitumor therapies. The advent of targeted immune therapies leading to successful outcomes in other malignancies has led to an increase in the number of clinical trials using these interventional strategies in patients with gynecological cancer. Generally, the role of immunotherapy is either to reactivate the immune response or to diminish the tumor-directed immune inhibition.

There are three stages of the dynamic process of immunoediting, also known as the three Es: an early elimination phase with the activation of an innate and adoptive immune response, an equilibrium phase where the isolated tumor cells are able to endure immune incursion, and an immune escape phase that the cancer cell variants can alter their genomic or antigenic phenotype or they are under the control of immunoregulatory phenomena to survive in the immunosuppressive medium. In order to activate tumor-directed immune responses, recent immune therapies have consisted of several approaches, including adoptive cell transfer (ACT), cancer vaccines, and immune checkpoint inhibitors.

Cervical cancer is unique among gynecologic malignant tumors because of its well-established and causative risk factor, chronic HPV infection. The infectious etiology of cervical cancer has led to effective vaccines for prevention; however, advanced stage/metastatic disease remains a principal cause of gynecologic cancer mortality in much of the world. The implementation of antiangiogenic therapy has greatly improved the treatment for relapsed/advanced disease over the last 5 years. Several clinical trials including CheckMate 358 and KEYNOTE-028 and KEYNOTE-158 are evaluating the role of immune checkpoint inhibitors in the treatment of cervical cancer.

In endometrial cancer, patients with advanced or disseminated recurrent disease have a poor prognosis, and most patients with peritoneal recurrence are considered incurable. Platinum and taxane chemotherapy produces response rates of 40–60%, which decreases to 20% for second-line drugs. So there is a need for development of more effective treatment for patients having advanced disease.

Approximately 25% of endometrial tumors are characterized by defects in the DNA mismatch repair system manifested by errors in DNA replication of trinucleotide repeat regions, commonly referred to as microsatellite instability. These defects in mismatch repair (MMR) also result in a high somatic mutation rate and accordingly increased number of neoantigens in these MMR-deficient tumors. In endometrial cancer, the presence of high microsatellite instability (MSI-H) has become an area of interest for use of immune checkpoint inhibitors.

For several reasons ovarian cancer is an ideal tumor type for which to consider an immunomodulatory management approach. Firstly, there is no negative impact of cancer itself on immunoregulatory cells that may be present within the bone marrow or other body locations. Secondly, while standard cytotoxic therapy of ovarian cancer can result in a depression in the number of immunoregulatory cell, these effects are generally modest in extent and short in duration. Lastly, it is common for patients with ovarian cancer to maintain a quite reasonable performance status and satisfactory nutrition.

A majority of ovarian cancer patients respond to cytotoxic chemotherapy and invariably are free from disease for periods varying from months to several years. This time interval can be exploited for required “activation” of immune defense mechanisms, either by using a tested vaccination strategy or any other form of immune modulation.

Multiple studies involving immune checkpoint inhibitors, conducted in advanced endometrial cancer, ovarian cancer, and cervical cancer, have shown promising preliminary results. But similar to that seen in other tumor types, continued work will need to focus on identifying those subsets of patients that will benefit from these therapies as these treatments are not without significant toxicities.

The immune system plays an important role in cancer pathogenesis. Numerous clinical trials and multiple researches dedicated to study therapies that involve the immune system to favorably impact the disease course in various malignancies have not only shown improved patient survival but also diversified the whole cancer management scenario by approval of the use of various immunotherapeutic agents in advanced malignancies [1].

Since cancer immunotherapy has emerged as an effective and appealing therapeutic option among other different therapeutic strategies and has been proven competent against multiple malignancies, it has led to an increase in research on immunomodulatory approaches in gynecological malignancies [2].

The ongoing research on the understanding of tumor biology and immunology has led to improved comprehension of mechanisms of immune recognition, regulation, and tumor escape that has provided new approaches for cancer immunotherapy [3].

2. Role of immune system in cancer

The principal role of the immune system is against foreign pathogens and infections. It is further classified as cellular and humoral immune systems, mediated by T and B lymphocytes and their products, respectively.

The initial innate immunity is nonspecific, and the adaptive immune response is the specialized defense. Both the strategies work in different manner. They employ the cellular immunity which has a rather fast response in eradicating intracellular microbes through the recognition of antigens, activation of antigen-presenting cells (APCs), and activation and proliferation of T cells. They also need humoral immunity mediated via antibodies produced by B cells for neutralizing toxins and act against infections. Where innate immunity works by releasing signals essential to stimulate responses from both T cells and B cells [4], the adaptive immune system is mainly consists of B cells, CD8+ cytotoxic T cells, as well as CD4+ helper T cell [5].

The immune system in tumor cells has a dynamic relationship, in which either it can identify or control tumor cells in a process called cancer immunosurveillance or cause tumor progression through chronic inflammation, immunoselection of poorly immunogenic variants, and suppressing antitumor immunity [6]. There are three stages of this dynamic process called immunoediting. The first is the elimination phase in which innate and adaptive immunity works together to identify and eliminate the cancer cells before they become clinically apparent [7]. If the cancer cells are not eliminated, they enter the second phase which is equilibrium. It can last from months to years. Here the cancer cells persist, but outgrowth is prevented by the immune system. Lastly the escape phase is in which either the cancer cell variants survive in the immunosuppressive microenvironment by altering genetic or antigenic phenotype or under the control of immunoregulatory phenomena. [8] In order to activate tumor-directed immune responses, recent immune therapies have consisted of several approaches, including adoptive cell transfer (ACT), cancer vaccines, and immune checkpoint inhibitors.

Gynecological cancers are a group of malignancies that involve different organs that comprise the female reproductive system. The most common types of gynecologic malignancies are cervical cancer, ovarian cancer, and endometrial cancer. Other less common gynecological malignancies arise from the vagina, vulva, and fallopian tubes [9].

3. Cervical cancer

Cervical cancer represents 6.6% of all female cancers. It is the fourth most common cancer in women with an estimated 570,000 new cases in 2018. Approximately 90% of deaths from cervical cancer occur in underdeveloped and developing countries [10]. Cervical cancer has emerged as a preventable disease due to currently employed screening tests which have highlighted HPV infection as an etiological factor. Although significant progress has been made in screening and prevention of cervical cancer, the 5-year overall survival remains 66% [11]. For cases diagnosed at an early stage, the recurrence rates vary between 10 and 20%, but for advanced cases, the rate of recurrence reaches up to 70% [12]. There is a need to improve outcomes, and immunotherapy could offer this possibility. The recognition of human papilloma virus as an etiological agent has greatly improved the understanding of the disease and led to improved strategies in prevention of cervical cancer [13]. The infectious etiology of cervical cancer has led to effective vaccines for prevention; however, advanced stage/metastatic disease remains a principal cause of gynecologic cancer mortality. Currently there are three licensed HPV prophylactic vaccines, namely, bivalent vaccine cervarix against HPV16/18, Gardasil against HPV-6/11/16/18, and Gardasil9, a nonavalent HPV-6/11/16/18/31/33/45/52/58 vaccine. All are based on on-infectious recombinant type-specific L1 capsid proteins assembled into viral-like particles (VLPs) as immunogens [14].

There is a huge unmet need for the treatment for women having advanced/recurrent cancer after standard chemotherapy and immunotherapy aims to fill that void, through therapies that harness a patient's own immune system to attack the cancer.

4. Cancer vaccines in cervical cancer

Cancer vaccines are used to mediate immune response by activating T cells which can specifically recognize cancer cells by tagging them with tumor-specific antigens E6 and E7. These antigen-tagged tumor cells are recognized by antigen-presenting cells and killed by cytotoxic T cells [15].

Live vector vaccines are highly immunogenic vaccines which can stimulate mucosal as well as humoral and/or cellular systemic immunity. They present E6 and E7 to APC to cause immune response through major histocompatibility complex MHC I [16]. Although they are attenuated vaccines, still care has to be taken before administering it in immunocompromised individuals. ADXS11-001 is a type of live attenuated vaccine that uses *Listeria monocytogenes* (Lm), a gram-positive intracellular bacterium as bacterial vector. It secretes HPV-16 E7 antigen fused to a nonhemolytic fragment of Lm protein listeriolysin O [17].

The following studies have been conducted (**Table 1**):

Study name	**Patient cohort**	**Treatment schedule**	**Response**	**Toxicity**
Maciag et al. [18] Phase I trial	*n* = 15 Recurrent or metastatic disease	DL1: ADXS11-001 1 × 109 two doses every 21 days DL2: ADXS11-001 3.3 × 109 two doses every 21 days DL3: ADXS11-001 1 × 1010 two doses every 21 days	Stable disease in 7 patients	Pyrexia (100%), vomiting 60%, pain (57%), chills, anemia (53%) Grade 3: 40% (6 pts)
Ghamande et al. [19] Phase I	*n* = 9 Recurrent or metastatic disease	DL1: ADXS11-001 5 × 109 thrice weekly during 12 weeks DL2: ADXS11-001 1 × 1010 thrice weekly during 12 weeks	—	TRAE: 75% AE: 99% Grade 1 and 2 Grade 3: chills, vomit, hypotension, tachycardia, fever, and nausea
Basu et al. [20] Phase II	*n* = 109 Advanced cervical cancer	Arm 1 ADXS11-001 monotherapy Arm 2 ADXS11-001 with cisplatin combination	Median progression-free survival (6.10 vs. 6.08 months) and the overall response rate (17.1% vs. 14.7%) were similar for both groups	More adverse effects in arm 2
Huh et al. [21] (GOG 0265) Phase II	*n* = 26 Recurrent or metastatic disease	ADXS11-001 1 × 109 every 28 days for 3 doses	Mean 12 months survival: 38.5% Median OS: 6.2 months	AE: 91% Grade 1 and 2 TRAE: 38%: nausea, vomiting, chills, fatigue, and fever

Table 1.
Role of vaccination in HPV-associated cervical cancer.

4.1 Peptide-based vaccines in cervical cancer

Refer **Table 2**.

Study name	Patient cohort	Treatment schedule	Response	Toxicity
Welters et al. [22] Phase II adjuvant	*n* = 6 Stage IB1 and HPV16+	HPV16 E6 E7 SLP vaccine	Vaccine-enhanced number and activity of HPV16-specific CD4+ and CD8+ cells	Grade 1 and Grade 2: local pain, fever, flu-like symptoms, swelling, itching, burning eyes
Poelgeest et al. [23] Phase II	*n* = 31 Recurrent or metastatic disease	HPV16 E6-E7 SLP vaccine 300 g for four doses every 21 day	Median OS: 12.6 months no tumor regression or delay of progression	Grade 1 and Grade 2: fever, fatigue, headache, flu-like symptoms, chills, nausea, swelling extremities, rash, vomiting, tingling extremities, and injection site pain

Table 2.
Peptide-based vaccine in cervical cancer.

4.2 Dendritic vaccines in cervical cancer

Refer **Table 3**.

Study name	Patient cohort	Treatment schedule	Response	Toxicity
Ramanathan et al. [24] Phase I	*n* = 14 Recurrent or metastatic disease	Arm 1: placebo three doses every 14 days Arm 2: unprimed DC three doses 1 × 106 cells every 14 days Arm 3: primed DC three doses 1 × 106 cells every 14 days	SD in Arm 3	Grade 1 and Grade 2: itching at injection site, fever, chills, abdominal discomfort, vomit, ALP increased
Ferrara et al. [25] Phase I	*n* = 15 Recurrent or metastatic disease	Analogous dendritic cells pulsed with HPV E7 protein	Serological response in 3 pts Cellular response in 4 pts No objective clinical response	
Santin et al. [26] Phase I	*n* = 10 Stage IB or IIA	DL1: HPV16/18 E7 antigen-pulsed DC5 × 106 for five doses every 21 days DL2: HPV16/18 E7 antigen-pulsed DC10 × 106 for five doses every 21 days DL3: HPV16/18 E7 antigen-pulsed DC15 × 106 for five doses every 21 days	CD4+ T-cell response in all patients	Mild swelling and erythema at the injection site

Table 3.
Dendritic vaccine in cervical cancer.

5. Immune checkpoint inhibitors in cervical cancer

5.1 PD1/PDL1 inhibitors

Programmed cell death protein-1/programmed death ligand-1 immunoregulatory axis is a promising target for cervical cancer treatment [27]. Pembrolizumab is a humanized monoclonal immunoglobulin G4 (IgG4) kappa isotype antibody targeting PD-1 (**Table 4**).

Other ongoing trials of pembrolizumab include PAPAYA Trial [30] which is a phase I study involving Stage Ib to Stage IV cervical cancer. The treatment schedule includes intravenous pembrolizumab followed by cisplatin-based chemoradiotherapy and brachytherapy and additional pembrolizumab after radiation. Another phase II trial with pembrolizumab followed by chemoradiotherapy and brachytherapy is also open for recruitment [31].

Nivolumab is a human IgG4 monoclonal antibody that causes stimulation of PD1 pathway-mediated immune response inhibition by binding to the PD-1 receptor and blocking its interaction with PD-L1 and PD-L2. [32] Checkmate 358 trial is a phase I/II trial by Hollebecque et al. in 19 patients of cervical cancer which studied nivolumab 240 mg every 2 weeks and showed ORR was 20.8% and disease control rate was 70.8%. Responses were observed regardless of PD-L1 expression, HPV status, and number of prior therapies [33].

Other trials of nivolumab include NRG-GY002, a phase II trial in recurrent or metastatic breast cancer [34]. A trial of nivolumab with HPV 16 SLp vaccine in HPV 16 positive cervical cancer is also underway [35].

Other checkpoint inhibitors under investigation include atezolizumab which is a fully humanized monoclonal antibody IgG1 isotype PD-L1. It is being studied to assess the safety and efficacy in combination with cyclophosphamide/carboplatin in gynecological cancer including cervical cancer in phase Ib PRO-LOG study [36]. Another phase II study is ongoing to study the synergistic action of antiangiogenic therapy with immunotherapy by combining bevacizumab with atezolizumab in women with recurrent or metastatic cervical cancer [37, 38],

Durvalumab is a human IgG1 monoclonal antibody that blocks the action of PD-L1 with PD1 and CD 80. It is being studied along with tremelimumab, which is an antibody against CTLA4 in patients who have failed to respond or relapsed to standard treatment [39].

5.2 CTLA-4 inhibitors

Ipilimumab is a fully human monoclonal IgG1κ antibody which acts against the cytotoxic T lymphocyte antigen-4 (CTLA-4). CTLA4 is an immune-inhibitory

Study name	Patient cohort	Treatment schedule	Response	Toxicity
Keynote 028 Frenel et al. [28] Phase Ib	*n* = 24 Patients having metastatic disease in PD L1 > =1%	Pembrolizumab 10 mg/kg every 2 weeks up to 2 years	ORR = 12.5% 6 months PFS 13% OS 66.7% (preliminary results)	75% pts with treatment-related adverse effects 20.8% with Grade 3 toxicity
Keynote 0158 Schellens et al. [29] Phase II	*n* = 47 Metastatic disease	Pembrolizumab 200 mg thrice weekly to 2 years	ORR 17% (independent of tumor PD L1 status)	Not reported

Table 4.
PD1/PDL1 inhibitors in cervical cancer.

Study name	Patient cohort	Treatment schedule	Response	Toxicity
Lheureux et al. [41] Phase I/II	*n* = 42 Recurrent or metastatic disease	Phase I: ipilimumab 3 mg/kg every 21 days for four doses Phase II: ipilimumab 10 mg/kg every 21 days for four doses and four cycles (same dose) every 12 weeks	Median PFS 2.5 months	Grade 3 toxicity: diarrhea, colitis
GOG9929 study Mayadev et al. [42] Phase I	*n* = 34 FIGO IB2/IIA or IIB/IIIB/IVA, positive nodes	Weekly cisplatin 40 mg/m^2 during 6 weeks and extended field radiotherapy. If no progression 2–6 weeks after DL1: ipilimumab 3 mg/kg for four doses every 21 days DL2: ipilimumab 10 mg/kg for four doses every 21 days DL3: ipilimumab 10 mg/kg for four doses every 21 days	1 year DFS 74%	Grade 1 and Grade 2: rash, endocrinopaties, gastrointestinal toxicity Grade 3: 16% including lipase increased, neutropenia, and rash

Table 5.
CTLA4 inhibitors in cervical cancer.

molecule which is expressed in activated T cells and in suppressor T regulatory cells [40] (**Table 5**).

5.3 Adoptive cell transfer therapy

Adoptive cell transfer therapy using autologous tumor-infiltrating lymphocytes is emerging as a promising treatment modality in immunotherapy for various cancers. There are two types of adoptive cell therapy which includes chimeric antigen receptor T-cell (CAR T-cell) therapy and tumor-infiltrating lymphocyte (TIL) therapy.

Chimeric antigen receptor (CAR) T-cell therapy involves genetically engineered patient's autologous T cells that causes them to express a CAR specific for a tumor antigen. These cells are extracted, further divided, and reinfused back into the patient [43].

A trial was conducted by Lu et al. which evaluated adoptive CD4+ T-cell therapy in solid metastatic cancer. It had two patients of metastatic cervical cancer, out of which one patient had objective complete response [44].

There is a trial ongoing to test the safety, feasibility, and efficacy of CAR T-cell immunotherapy in patients who have GD@, PSMA, Muc1, mesothelin, or positive cervical cancer markers by Chang et al. [45].

TIL therapy predates the CAR T-cell therapy, and the basic principle involves the ex vivo culture of tumor specimens which have been resected and expansion of tumor-infiltrating lymphocytes (TILs) with interleukin-2. Selected T cells of a preferred antigen specificity and phenotype can be identified in vitro and divided. The number of antigen-specific T cells in peripheral blood after this method usually exceeds by far that possible by current vaccine treatment strategies alone. In addition, adoptive T cells appear more effective in inducing tumor regression than lymphocytes generated by vaccines, suggesting greater ability to overcome tumor-mediated immune evasion mechanisms [46].

Stevanovic et al. [47] conducted a trial on 17 patients of metastatic cervical cancer who received high-dose lymphocyte-depleting chemotherapy followed by aldesleukin. Patients were treated with a single infusion of human papillomavirus (HPV) E6 and E7 reactivity (HPV-TILs). Three of nine patients experienced objective tumor responses (two complete responses and one partial response).

6. Endometrial cancer

Endometrial cancer is the 4th most commonly occurring cancer in women and the 15th most commonly occurring cancer overall. There were over 380,000 new cases in 2018 [48]. In women with advanced and recurrent cancer, the prognosis is considered very poor. Unfortunately, there are limited treatment options for advanced or recurrent endometrioid endometrial cancer. However, with the advent of immunotherapy, immune checkpoint inhibitors have shown promising results in these cases.

Study name	Patient cohort	Treatment schedule	Response	Toxicity
Ott et al. [53]	*n* = 24 Locally advanced or metastatic PD-L1-positive endometrial cancer	Pembrolizumab 10 mg/kg every 2 weeks for up to 24 months or until progression or unacceptable toxicity	Three (13%) patients achieved confirmed partial response. Three additional patients achieved stable disease, with a median duration of 24.6 weeks	Grade 3 treatment-related AEs were reported in four patients
Makker et al. [54] Phase II	*n* = 53 Metastatic endometrial cancer unselected for microsatellite instability or PD-L1	20 mg oral lenvatinib daily plus 200 mg intravenous pembrolizumab every 3 weeks, until progression or unacceptable toxicity	Patients had an objective response at week 24	Serious treatment-related adverse events occurred in 16 (30%) patients, and one treatment-related death was reported (intracranial hemorrhage)
Santin et al. [55]	*n* = 2 Pretreated polymerase ε (POLE) ultramutated and MSH6 hypermutated recurrent endometrial tumors refractory to surgery, radiation, and chemotherapy	Anti-PD1 immune checkpoint inhibitor nivolumab 3 mg/kg biweekly	Both patients demonstrated a remarkable clinical response to the anti-PD1 immune checkpoint inhibitor nivolumab	No Grade 3 or higher side effects reported
Fleming et al. [56]	*n* = 15 Previously treated recurrent endometrial cancer	Atezolizumab 1200 mg or 15 mg/kg IV q3w was administered until toxicity or loss of clinical benefit	ORR was 13% (2/15) Of the remaining pts, two had SD, nine had PD, and two were non-evaluable	Seven (47%) pts had any related AE, mainly G1-2 (5 pts). No G4-5-related AEs occurred

Table 6.
Immunotherapy in endometrial cancer.

Microsatellite instability-high (MSI-H) status, tumor mutation burden, and high PD-L1 expression have been associated with higher response rates to this therapy [49].

Approximately 25% of endometrial cancer show microsatellite instability which is caused by defects in mismatch repair genes. These defective MMR genes lead to high somatic mutation rates, thereby increasing the number of neoantigens in MMR-deficient tumors [50].

Endometrial cancer has been subdivided into four prognostically distinct molecular subgroups based on the findings of the cancer genome atlas, namely, polymerase epsilon (*POLE*) ultramutated, MSI hypermutated, copy-number (CN) low, and CN high [51].

The ultramutated POLE subgroup and MSI hypermutated subgroup have immune-rich microenvironment and high mutation load. Evidence has supported over-expression of the PD-1/PD-L1 pathway in these molecular subtypes, and therefore, PD1/PD L1-targeted immunotherapy has a role in these tumors [52] (**Table 6**).

An ongoing phase II, two group trials are studying the role of avelumab in POLE-mutated endometrial cancer and MSS-mutated endometrial cancer. Avelumab is administered at 10 mg/kg as 1-hour IV infusion every 2 weeks until disease progression or unacceptable toxicity. Sixteen patients are enrolled in each cohort in the first stage. The preliminary results are yet to be published [57].

6.1 Anticancer vaccines in endometrial cancer

The following studies have been conducted (**Table 7**).

7. Ovarian cancer

Ovarian cancer accounts for 2.5% of all malignancies among females but 5% of female cancer deaths because of low survival rates, largely driven by late-stage diagnoses [60]. There were nearly 300,000 new cases in 2018. Ovarian cancer is considered to be an ideal type of tumor which can be dealt with immunomodulatory

Study name	Patient cohort	Treatment schedule	Response	Toxicity
Ohno et al. [58], phase II	$n = 12$ WT1/human leukocyte antigen (HLA)-A*2402-positive gynecological cancer	Intradermal injections of a HLA-A*2402-restricted, modified 9-mer WT1 peptide every week for 12 weeks	Stable disease in three patients and progressive disease in nine patients. The disease control rate was 25.0%	Local erythema occurred at the WT1 vaccine injection site
Coosemans et al. [59]	$n = 6$ Pretreated patients with uterine cancer	Four times weekly vaccines of autologous dendritic cells (DCs) electroporated with WT1 mRNA	Three out of four human leucocyte antigen-A2 (HLA-A2)-positive patients showed an oncological response. Two HLA-A2-negative patients did not show an oncological or an immunological response	One patient had a local allergic reaction

Table 7.
Anticancer vaccines in endometrial cancer.

approach as the disease does not negatively affect the immunoregulatory cells in the bone marrow or other locations of the body, and the patients suffering from ovarian cancer maintain a relatively good performance status even in later stages, so immunotherapy can be used as a potential treatment option in these patients. Cytotoxic chemotherapy given in ovarian cancer can negatively impact the immunoregulatory cells, but the effect is short lasting. Further the patients who are in advanced stages, if they respond to standard treatment of ovarian cancer, have a relatively long disease-free period which is substantial for the activation of immune defense mechanism either by cancer vaccines or by immunomodulator drugs [61].

7.1 Immune checkpoint inhibitors in ovarian cancer

The first published data supporting checkpoint inhibitors as a potentially valuable therapeutic option in ovarian cancer were observed in the trials of the anti-PD-1 antibody nivolumab and the anti-PD-L1 antibody BMS-93655 [62]. Other studies are as follows (**Table 8**).

Study name	Patient cohort	Treatment schedule	Response	Toxicity
Hamanishi et al. [63] Phase II	*n* = 20 Platinum-resistant ovarian cancer	IV nivolumab every 2 weeks at a dose of 1 or 3 mg/kg	Overall response rate was 15%, and the disease control rate was 45%	Grade 3 or 4 TRAE in 40% patients
Disis et al. [64] Phase Ib	*n* = 124 Recurrent/refractory ovarian cancer	Avelumab 10 mg/kg IV every 2 weeks	ORR was 9.7% based on 12 partial responses; 6 were ongoing. Stable disease was observed in 55 pts (44.4%); disease control rate was 54.0%	Grade 3 or 4 TRAEs were reported in 6.5%
Varga et al. [65] Phase Ib	*n* = 26 Advanced ovarian cancer	Pembrolizumab 10 mg/kg was given every 2 weeks for up to 2 years or until confirmed progression or unacceptable toxicity	The best overall (confirmed) response was 11.5%. 6/26 (23.1%) had evidence of tumor reduction; 3 had a tumor reduction of at least 30%	Drug-related AEs occurred in 69.2% of pts
Lee et al. [66] Phase I/II	*n* = 12 BRCA positive with ovarian cancer	Durvalumab at 1500 mg every 4 weeks plus olaparib at 300 mg twice daily and durvalumab at 1500 mg every 4 weeks plus cediranib at 20 mg 5 days on/2 days off per week	ORR of 17% and disease control rate of 83%	Grade 3 or 4 TRAEs were reported in 75% patients

Table 8.
Immune checkpoint inhibitors in ovarian cancer.

Ongoing trials include JAVELIN Ovarian 200 is the first phase III trial, which is a three-arm trial, comparing avelumab administered alone or in combination with pegylated liposomal doxorubicin versus pegylated liposomal doxorubicin alone in patients with platinum-resistant/refractory recurrent ovarian cancer [67].

NCT02839707 is undergoing trial which is comparing pegylated liposomal doxorubicin with atezolizumab and/or bevacizumab in refractory ovarian cancer [68].

A phase II study by Wenham et al. [69] is studying combination of weekly paclitaxel and an anti-PD-1 (pembrolizumab). The primary endpoint of this study is a 6-month progression-free survival rate.

ATALANTE trial is an ongoing phase III study to assess the efficacy of atezolizumab in combination with platinum-based chemotherapy plus bevacizumab administered concurrent to chemotherapy and in maintenance [70].

CheckMate 032 study trial to study the safety and efficacy of nivolumab as a single agent or in combination with ipilimumab is currently underway [71].

Similar trial in which nivolumab with or without ipilimumab in treating patients with persistent or recurrent epithelial ovarian is being studied by the National Cancer Institute [72].

A phase II trial to determine the median immune-related progression-free survival (irPFS) in combination of an anti-CTLA-4 antibody (tremelimumab) with an anti-PD-L1 antibody (durvalumab) versus their sequential use in platinum-resistant epithelial ovarian cancer is also currently ongoing [73].

Multiple other trial are using immune checkpoint inhibitors in initial therapy to improve progression-free survival like durvalumab or pembrolizumab with standard paclitaxel and carboplatin therapy, where pembrolizumab is used as adjuvant therapy after surgery [74]. The role of immune checkpoint inhibitors as maintenance therapy is also under investigation with JAVELIN Ovarian 100 phase II study of avelumab (anti-PD-L1) as maintenance after standard therapy or in combination with standard therapy and then continued as maintenance treatment [75].

7.2 Cancer vaccines in ovarian cancer

Various types of cancer vaccines are studied for the treatment of ovarian cancer.

The cancer testis antigen, NY ESO1, is most frequently expressed in epithelial ovarian cancer, and vaccine against it has shown induced T-cell-specific immunogenicity [76]. Since NY-ESO-1 is regulated by DNA methylation, it was hypothesized that DNA methyltransferase (DNMT) inhibitors may augment NY-ESO-1 vaccine therapy. Decitabine is a hypomethylating agent that inhibits DNA methyltransferase. A phase I trial was conducted to study dose escalation of decitabine in addition to NY-ESO-1 vaccine and doxorubicin liposome in 12 patients with relapsed epithelial ovarian carcinoma. The results showed stable disease or partial response in six patients [77].

Sabbatini et al. conducted a phase I trial in 28 patients which showed that in order to enhance the immunogenic response to NY-ESO1, the addition of immune modulation agents to the vaccine preparation such as Montanide and immunostimulants such as the toll-like receptor (TLR) ligand poly-ICLC (polyinosinic-polycytidylic acid—stabilized by lysine and carboxymethylcellulose) can be considered [78].

Other antigen under investigation is Her/neu2, which is expressed in 90% of epithelial ovarian cancers. A phase I/II study conducted BY Chu et al. demonstrated a 90% 3-year overall survival response in patients with advanced ovarian cancer who were remission for vaccination with monocyte-derived dendritic cells (DC) loaded with Her2/neu, hTERT, and PADRE peptides, with or without low-dose intravenous cyclophosphamide [79].

In a phase I/II study by Baek et al., 10 ovarian cancer patients with minimal residual disease were treated with dendritic cell vaccination with IL2. Three out of 10 patients showed maintenance of complete response, and one patient showed stable disease [80].

A phase II study was conducted to study the efficacy of personalized peptide vaccine (PPV) for recurrent ovarian cancer patients by Kawano et al. [81]. The patients enrolled in this study showed an overall survival (OS) of 39.3 months in platinum-sensitive cases and 16.2 months in platinum-resistant cases. This was attributed to be secondary to the stabilization of disease and the prolongation of tumor progression rather than disease regression.

7.3 Adoptive cell transfer in ovarian cancer

Adoptive cell transfer therapy is not widely studied in ovarian cancers. In a Japanese study by Fujita et al., 13 patients with epithelial ovarian cancer were treated with tumor-infiltrating lymphocyte therapy. Eleven patients served as control group who received only chemotherapy following primary operation. The estimated 3-year overall survival rate of disease-free patients in the TIL group and in the control group was 100 and 67.5%, respectively [82].

Vulvar and vaginal cancer: Immunotherapy has shown promising results in advanced gynecological cancer. Checkmate 358 trial has shown that nivolumab has encouraging clinical activity in cases of HPV-positive vulvar and vaginal malignancies. A lot of research is warranted to establish immunotherapy as emerging treatment option in these cancers.

8. Conclusion

Immunotherapy is emerging as a viable treatment modality in multiple cancers, and its safety and efficacy are under investigation in advanced gynecological malignancies. Immune checkpoint inhibitors have shown promising preliminary results in advanced ovarian, cervical, and endometrial cancer.

Author details

Neha Sharma[1] and Deepti Sharma[2*]

1 Department of Radiation Oncology, Lady Hardinge Medical College and Associated SSK and KSC Hospital, New Delhi, India

2 Department of Radiation Oncology, Institute of Liver and Biliary Science, New Delhi, India

*Address all correspondence to: drdeeptisharma16@gmail.com

References

[1] Borghaei H, Smith MR, Campbell KS. Immunotherapy of cancer. European Journal of Pharmacology. 2009;**625**:41-54

[2] Jazaeri A, Coleman RL, Sood AK, Frumovitz MM, Soliman PT, Shafer A, et al. A practical guide for the safe implementation of early phase drug development and immunotherapy program in gynecologic oncology practice. Gynecologic Oncology. 2018;**151**:374-380

[3] Ito F, Chang AE. Cancer immunotherapy. Surgical Oncology Clinics of North America. 2013;**22**:765-783

[4] Woo S-R, Corrales L, Gajewski TF. Innate immune recognition of cancer. Annual Review of Immunology. 2015;**33**:445-474

[5] Binder RJ. Functions of heat shock proteins in pathways of the innate and adaptive immune system. The Journal of Immunology. 2014;**193**:5765-5771

[6] Zhang H, Chen J. Current status and future directions of cancer immunotherapy. Journal of Cancer. 2018;**9**:1773-1781

[7] Vesely MD, Schreiber RD. Cancer immunoediting: Antigens, mechanisms, and implications to cancer immunotherapy. Annals of the New York Academy of Sciences. 2013;**1284**:1-5

[8] Shore ND. Advances in the understanding of cancer immunotherapy. BJU International. 2015;**116**:321-329

[9] Maheshwari A, Kumar N, Mahantshetty U. Gynecological cancers: A summary of published Indian data. South Asian Journal of Cancer. 2016;**5**:112

[10] Vu M, Yu J, Awolude OA, Chuang L. Cervical cancer worldwide. Current Problems in Cancer. 2018;**42**:457-465

[11] Cervical Cancer—Statistics [Internet]. Cancer.Net. 2019. Available from: https://www.cancer.net/cancer-types/cervical-cancer/statistics

[12] Friedlander M, Grogan M, US Preventative Services Task Force. Guidelines for the treatment of recurrent and metastatic cervical cancer. The Oncologist. 2002;**7**(4):342-347

[13] Schiffman M, Wentzensen N, Wacholder S, Kinney W, Gage JC, Castle PE. Human papillomavirus testing in the prevention of cervical cancer. Journal of the National Cancer Institute. 2011;**103**:368-383

[14] Pinto LA, Dillner J, Beddows S, Unger ER. Immunogenicity of HPV prophylactic vaccines: Serology assays and their use in HPV vaccine evaluation and development. Vaccine. 2018;**36**(32):4792-4799. DOI: 10.1016/j.vaccine.2017.11.089

[15] Miles B, Safran HP, Monk BJ. Therapeutic options for treatment of human papillomavirus-associated cancers—Novel immunologic vaccines: ADXS11-001. Gynecologic Oncology Research and Practice. 2017;**4**:10

[16] Silva AJD, Zangirolami TC, Novo-Mansur MTM, Giordano RDC, Martins EAL. Live bacterial vaccine vectors: An overview. Brazilian Journal of Microbiology. 2014;**45**:1117-1129

[17] Pan Z-K, Ikonomidis G, Lazenby A, Pardoll D, Paterson Y. A recombinant *Listeria monocytogenes* vaccine expressing a model tumour antigen protects mice against lethal tumour cell challenge and causes regression of established tumours. Nature Medicine. 1995;**1**:471-477

[18] Maciag PC, Radulovic S, Rothman J. The first clinical use of a live-attenuated Listeria monocytogenes vaccine: A phase I safety study of Lm-LLO-E7 in patients with advanced carcinoma of the cervix. Vaccine. 2009;**27**(30):3975-3983

[19] Ghamande SA, Platt D, Wheatley D, Rungruang BJ, Janik JE, Khleif S. Phase I study evaluating high-dose treatment with ADXS11-001, a *Listeria monocytogenes*-listeriolysin O (Lm-LLO) immunotherapy, in women with cervical cancer. Journal of Clinical Oncology. 2016;**34**(15 Suppl.):e14580

[20] Basu P, Mehta A, Jain M, Gupta S, Nagarkar RV, John S, et al. A randomized phase 2 study of ADXS11-001 *Listeria monocytogenes*–Listeriolysin O immunotherapy with or without cisplatin in treatment of advanced cervical cancer. International Journal of Gynecologic Cancer. 2018;**28**:764-772

[21] Huh WK, Brady WE, Moore KN, Lankes HA, Monk BJ, Aghajanian C, et al. A phase 2 study of live-attenuated listeria monocytogenes cancer immunotherapy (ADXS11-001) in the treatment of persistent or recurrent cancer of the cervix (GOG-0265). Journal of Clinical Oncology. 2014;**32** (15 suppl.):TPS5617

[22] Welters MJ, Kenter GG, Piersma SJ, Vloon AP, Lowik MJ, DMB-VD M, et al. Induction of tumor-specific CD4 and CD8 T-cell immunity in cervical cancer patients by a human papillomavirus type 16 E6 and E7 long peptides vaccine. Clinical Cancer Research. 2008;**14**:178-187

[23] Poelgeest MIEV, Welters MJP, Esch EMGV, Stynenbosch LFM, Kerpershoek G, Van Meerten ELVP, et al. HPV16 synthetic long peptide (HPV16-SLP) vaccination therapy of patients with advanced or recurrent HPV16-induced gynecological carcinoma, a phase II trial. Journal of Translational Medicine. 2013;**11**:88

[24] Ramanathan P, Ganeshrajah S, Raghanvan RK, Singh SS, Thangarajan R. Development and clinical evaluation of dendritic cell vaccines for HPV related cervical cancer—A feasibility study. Asian Pacific Journal of Cancer Prevention. 2014;**15**:5909-5916

[25] Ferrara A, Nonn M, Sehr P, Schreckenberger C, Pawlita M, Dürst M, et al. Dendritic cell-based tumor vaccine for cervical cancer II: Results of a clinical pilot study in 15 individual patients. Journal of Cancer Research and Clinical Oncology. 2003;**129**:521-530

[26] Santin AD, Bellone S, Palmieri M, Zanolini A, Ravaggi A, Siegel ER, et al. Human papillomavirus type 16 and 18 E7-pulsed dendritic cell vaccination of stage IB or IIA cervical cancer patients: A phase I escalating-dose trial. Journal of Virology. 2007;**82**:1968-1979

[27] Reddy OL, Shintaku PI, Moatamed NA. Programmed death-ligand 1 (PD-L1) is expressed in a significant number of the uterine cervical carcinomas. Diagnostic Pathology. 2017;**12**:45

[28] Frenel J-S, Tourneau CL, O'neil BH, Ott PA, Piha-Paul SA, Gomez-Roca CA, et al. Pembrolizumab in patients with advanced cervical squamous cell cancer: Preliminary results from the phase Ib KEYNOTE-028 study. Journal of Clinical Oncology. 2016;**34**:5515

[29] Schellens JH, Marabelle A, Zeigenfuss S, Ding J, Pruit S, Chung H. Pembrolizumab for previously treated advanced cervical squamous cell cancer: preliminary results from the phase 2 KEYNOTE-158 study. Journal of Clinical Oncology. 2017;**35**(15 Suppl):5514

[30] A Study of Pembrolizumab and Platinum with Radiotherapy in Cervix Cancer - Full Text View - ClinicalTrials.gov, clinicaltrials.gov/ct2/show/NCT03144466

[31] Pembrolizumab and Chemoradiation Treatment for Advanced Cervical Cancer—Full Text View [Internet]. ClinicalTrials.gov. Available from: https://clinicaltrials.gov/ct2/show/NCT02635360

[32] Guo L, Zhang H, Chen B. Nivolumab as programmed death-1 (PD-1) inhibitor for targeted immunotherapy in tumor. Journal of Cancer. 2017;**8**:410-416

[33] Hollebecque A, Meyer T, Moore KN, Machiels J-PH, De Greve J, López-Picazo J. An open-label, multicohort, phase I/II study of nivolumab in patients with virus-associated tumors (CheckMate 358): Efficacy and safety in recurrent or metastatic (R/M) cervical, vaginal, and vulvar cancers. Journal of Clinical Oncology 2017;**35**(15 Suppl.):5504

[34] Nivolumab in Treating Patients With Persistent, Recurrent, or Metastatic Cervical Cancer—Full Text View [Internet]. ClinicalTrials.gov. Available from: https://clinicaltrials.gov/ct2/show/NCT02257528

[35] Nivolumab and HPV-16 Vaccination in Patients With HPV-16 Positive Incurable Solid Tumors—Full Text View [Internet]. ClinicalTrials.gov. Available from: https://clinicaltrials.gov/ct2/show/NCT02426892

[36] Carboplatin-cyclophosphamide Combined With Atezolizumab—Full Text View [Internet]. ClinicalTrials.gov. Available from: https://clinicaltrials.gov/ct2/show/NCT02914470

[37] Atezolizumab and Bevacizumab in Treating Patients With Recurrent, Persistent, or Metastatic Cervical Cancer—Full Text View [Internet]. ClinicalTrials.gov. Available from: https://clinicaltrials.gov/ct2/show/NCT02921269

[38] Shrimali RK, Yu Z, Theoret MR, Chinnasamy D, Restifo NP, Rosenberg SA. Antiangiogenic agents can increase lymphocyte infiltration into tumor and enhance the effectiveness of adoptive immunotherapy of cancer. Cancer Research. 2010;**70**:6171-6180

[39] A Phase 1 Study to Evaluate MEDI4736 in Combination With Tremelimumab—Full Text View [Internet]. ClinicalTrials.gov. Available from: https://clinicaltrials.gov/ct2/show/NCT01975831

[40] Graziani G, Tentori L, Navarra P. Ipilimumab: A novel immunostimulatory monoclonal antibody for the treatment of cancer. Pharmacological Research. 2012;**65**:9-22

[41] Lheureux S, Butler M, Fleming G, Hirte H, Cristea M, Ghatage P, et al. 938TiPA phase 1/2 study of ipilimumab in women with metastatic or recurrent hpv-related cervical carcinoma: A study of the princess margaret and Chicago N01 Consortia. Annals of Oncology. 2014;**25**:iv324

[42] Mayadev J, Brady WE, Lin YG, Silva DMD, Lankes HA, Fracasso PM, et al. A phase I study of sequential ipilimumab in the definitive treatment of node positive cervical cancer: GOG 9929. Journal of Clinical Oncology. 2017;**35**:5526

[43] Miliotou AN, Papadopoulou LC. CAR T-cell therapy: A new era in cancer immunotherapy. Current Pharmaceutical Biotechnology. 2018;**19**:5-18

[44] Lu Y-C, Parker LL, Lu T, Zheng Z, Toomey MA, White DE, et al. Treatment of patients with metastatic cancer using a major histocompatibility complex class II–restricted T-cell receptor targeting the cancer germline antigen MAGE-A3. Journal of Clinical Oncology. 2017;**35**:3322-3329

[45] Intervention of CAR-T Against Cervical Cancer—Full Text View

[Internet]. ClinicalTrials.gov. Available from: https://clinicaltrials.gov/ct2/show/NCT03356795

[46] Zsiros E, Tsuji T, Odunsi K. Adoptive T-cell therapy is a promising salvage approach for advanced or recurrent metastatic cervical cancer. Journal of Clinical Oncology. 2015;**33**:1521-1522

[47] Stevanović S, Draper LM, Langhan MM, Campbell TE, Kwong ML, Wunderlich JR, et al. Complete regression of metastatic cervical cancer after treatment with human papillomavirus–targeted tumor-infiltrating T cells. Journal of Clinical Oncology. 2015;**33**(14):1543-1550

[48] Endometrial cancer statistics [Internet]. World Cancer Research Fund. 2018. Available from: https://www.wcrf.org/dietandcancer/cancer-trends/endometrial-cancer-statistics

[49] Zhao P, Li L, Jiang X, Li Q. Mismatch repair deficiency/microsatellite instability-high as a predictor for anti-PD-1/PD-L1 immunotherapy efficacy. Journal of Hematology & Oncology. 2019;**12**

[50] Alexandrov LB, Nik-Zainal S, Wedge DC, Campbell PJ, Stratton MR. Deciphering signatures of mutational processes operative in human cancer. Cell Reports. 2013;**3**:246-259

[51] Levine DA. Integrated genomic characterization of endometrial carcinoma. Nature. 2013;**497**(7447): 67-73. DOI: 10.1038/nature12113

[52] Gargiulo P et al. Tumor genotype and immune microenvironment in POLE-ultramutated and MSI-hypermutated endometrial cancers: New candidates for checkpoint blockade immunotherapy? Cancer Treatment Reviews. 2016;**48**:61-68. DOI: 10.1016/j.ctrv.2016.06.008

[53] Ott PA, Bang Y-J, Berton-Rigaud D, Elez E, Pishvaian MJ, Rugo HS, et al. Safety and antitumor activity of pembrolizumab in advanced programmed death ligand 1–positive endometrial cancer: Results from the KEYNOTE-028 study. Journal of Clinical Oncology. 2017;**35**:2535-2541

[54] Makker V, Rasco D, Vogelzang NJ, Brose MS, Cohn AL, Mier J, et al. Lenvatinib plus pembrolizumab in patients with advanced endometrial cancer: An interim analysis of a multicentre, open-label, single-arm, phase 2 trial. The Lancet Oncology. 2019;**20**:711-718

[55] Santin AD, Bellone S, Buza N, Choi J, Schwartz PE, Schlessinger J, et al. Regression of chemotherapy-resistant polymerase (POLE) ultra-mutated and MSH6 hyper-mutated endometrial tumors with nivolumab. Clinical Cancer Research. 2016;**22**:5682-5687. DOI: 10.1158/1078-0432.ccr-16-1031

[56] Fleming GF, Emens LA, Eder JP, Hamilton EP, Liu JF, Liu B, et al. Clinical activity, safety and biomarker results from a phase Ia study of atezolizumab (atezo) in advanced/recurrent endometrial cancer (rEC). Journal of Clinical Oncology. 2017;**35**:5585. DOI: 10.1200/jco.2017.35.15_suppl.5585

[57] Konstantinopoulos P, Liu J, Barry W, Krasner C, Buss M, Birrer M, et al. Phase II, two-stage study of avelumab in patients with microsatellite stable (MSS), microsatellite instable (MSI) and polymerase epsilon (POLE) mutated recurrent or persistent endometrial cancer. Gynecologic Oncology. 2018;**149**:24-25. DOI: 10.1016/j.ygyno.2018.04.060

[58] Ohno S, Kyo S, Myojo S, Dohi S, Ishizaki J, Miyamoto K, et al. Wilms' tumor 1 (WT1) peptide immunotherapy for gynecological malignancy. Anticancer Research. 2009;**29**:4779-4784

[59] Coosemans A, Vanderstraeten A, Tuyaerts S, Verschuere T, Moerman P, Berneman ZN, et al. Wilms' tumor gene 1 (WT1)-loaded dendritic cell immunotherapy in patients with uterine tumors: A phase I/II clinical trial. Anticancer Research. 2013;**33**:5495-5500

[60] Howlader N, Noone AM, Krapcho M, et al., editors. SEER Cancer Statistics Review, 1975-2014. Bethesda, MD: National Cancer Institute; 2017. Available from: seer.cancer.gov/csr/1975_2014/. [Accessed: 01 March 2018]

[61] Markman M. Immunotherapy in ovarian cancer—where are we going? American Journal of Hematology/Oncology. 2016. Available from: https://www.gotoper.com/publications/ajho/2016/2016feb/immunotherapy-in-ovarian-cancer-where-are-we-going

[62] Taneja SS. Re: safety and activity of anti-PD-L1 antibody in patients with advanced cancer. Journal of Urology. 2012;**188**:2148-2149

[63] Hamanishi J, Mandai M, Ikeda T, Minami M, Kawaguchi A, Murayama T, et al. Safety and antitumor activity of anti-PD-1 antibody, nivolumab, in patients with platinum-resistant ovarian cancer. Journal of Clinical Oncology. 2015;**33**:4015-4022

[64] Disis ML, Patel MR, Pant S, Hamilton EP, Lockhart AC, Kelly K, et al. Avelumab (MSB0010718C; anti-PD-L1) in patients with recurrent/refractory ovarian cancer from the JAVELIN solid tumor phase Ib trial: Safety and clinical activity. Journal of Clinical Oncology. 2016;**34**:5533

[65] Varga A, Piha-Paul SA, Ott PA, Mehnert JM, Berton-Rigaud D, Johnson EA, et al. Antitumor activity and safety of pembrolizumab in patients (pts) with PD-L1 positive advanced ovarian cancer: Interim results from a phase Ib study. Journal of Clinical Oncology. 2015;**33**:5510

[66] Lee JM et al. Safety and clinical activity of the programmed death-ligand 1 inhibitor durvalumab in combination with poly (ADP-ribose) polymerase inhibitor olaparib or vascular endothelial growth factor receptor 1-3 inhibitor cediranib in women's cancers: A dose-escalation, phase I study. Journal of Clinical Oncology. 2017;**35**(19):2193-2202

[67] Pujade-Lourraine E, Colombo N, Disis ML, Fujiwara K, Ledermann JA, Mirza MR, et al. Avelumab (MSB0010718C; anti-PD-L1) ± pegylated liposomal doxorubicin vs pegylated liposomal doxorubicin alone in patients with platinum-resistant/refractory ovarian cancer: The phase III JAVELIN Ovarian 200 trial. Journal of Clinical Oncology. 2016;**34**(15 suppl.):TPS5600

[68] Pegylated Liposomal Doxorubicin Hydrochloride With Atezolizumab and/or Bevacizumab in Treating Patients With Recurrent Ovarian, Fallopian Tube, or Primary Peritoneal Cancer—Full Text View [Internet]. ClinicalTrials.gov. Available from: https://clinicaltrials.gov/ct2/show/NCT02839707

[69] Wenham RM, Apte SM, Shahzad MM, Lee JK, Dorman D, Chon HS. Phase II trial of dose dense (weekly) paclitaxel with pembrolizumab (MK-3475) in platinum-resistant recurrent ovarian cancer. Journal of Clinical Oncology. 2016;**34**(15 suppl.):TPS5612

[70] ATALANTE: Atezolizumab vs Placebo Phase III Study in Late Relapse Ovarian Cancer Treated With Chemotherapy Bevacizumab—Full Text View [Internet]. ClinicalTrials.gov. Available from: https://clinicaltrials.gov/ct2/show/NCT02891824

[71] A Study of Nivolumab by Itself or Nivolumab Combined With Ipilimumab in Patients With Advanced or Metastatic Solid Tumors—Full Text View

[Internet]. ClinicalTrials.gov. Available from: https://clinicaltrials.gov/ct2/show/NCT01928394

[72] Nivolumab With or Without Ipilimumab in Treating Patients With Persistent or Recurrent Epithelial Ovarian, Primary Peritoneal, or Fallopian Tube Cancer—Full Text View [Internet]. ClinicalTrials.gov. Available from: https://clinicaltrials.gov/ct2/show/NCT02498600

[73] Durvalumab and Tremelimumab in Treating Participants With Recurrent or Refractory Ovarian, Primary Peritoneal, or Fallopian Tube Cancer—Full Text View [Internet]. ClinicalTrials.gov. Available from: https://clinicaltrials.gov/ct2/show/NCT03026062

[74] Pembrolizumab, Carboplatin, and Paclitaxel in Treating Patients With Stage III-IV Ovarian, Primary Peritoneal, or Fallopian Tube Cancer—Full Text View [Internet]. ClinicalTrials.gov. Available from: https://clinicaltrials.gov/ct2/show/NCT02520154

[75] Avelumab in Previously Untreated Patients With Epithelial Ovarian Cancer (JAVELIN OVARIAN 100)—Full Text View [Internet]. ClinicalTrials.gov. Available from: https://clinicaltrials.gov/ct2/show/NCT02718417

[76] Diefenbach CS, Gnjatic S, Sabbatini P, Aghajanian C, Hensley ML, Spriggs DR, et al. Safety and immunogenicity study of NY-ESO-1b peptide and montanide ISA-51 vaccination of patients with epithelial ovarian cancer in high-risk first remission. Clinical Cancer Research. 2008;**14**:2740-2748

[77] Odunsi K, Matsuzaki J, James SR, Mhawech-Fauceglia P, Tsuji T, Miller A, et al. Epigenetic potentiation of NY-ESO-1 vaccine therapy in human ovarian cancer. Cancer Immunology Research. 2014. Available from: https://www.ncbi.nlm.nih.gov/pubmed/24535937

[78] Sabbatini P, Tsuji T, Ferran L, Ritter E, Sedrak C, Tuballes K, et al. Phase I trial of overlapping long peptides from a tumor self-antigen and poly-ICLC shows rapid induction of integrated immune response in ovarian cancer patients. Clinical Cancer Research. 2012. Available from: https://www.ncbi.nlm.nih.gov/pubmed/23032745

[79] Chu CS, Boyer J, Schullery DS, Gimotty PA, Gamerman V, Bender J, et al. Phase I/II randomized trial of dendritic cell vaccination with or without cyclophosphamide for consolidation therapy of advanced ovarian cancer in first or second remission. Cancer Immunology, Immunotherapy. 2012. Available from: https://www.ncbi.nlm.nih.gov/pubmed/22021066

[80] Baek S, Kim Y-M, Kim S-B, Kim C-S, Kwon S-W, Kim YM, et al. Therapeutic DC vaccination with IL-2 as a consolidation therapy for ovarian cancer patients: A phase I/II trial [Internet]. Cellular & Molecular Immunology. 2015 Available from: https://www.ncbi.nlm.nih.gov/pubmed/24976269

[81] Kawano K, Tsuda N, Matsueda S, Sasada T, Watanabe N, Ushijima K, et al. Feasibility study of personalized peptide vaccination for recurrent ovarian cancer patients. Immunopharmacology and Immunotoxicology. 2014. Available from: https://www.ncbi.nlm.nih.gov/pubmed/24773550

[82] Fujita K, Ikarashi H, Takakuwa K, Kodama S, Tokunaga A, Takahashi T, et al. Prolonged disease-free period in patients with advanced epithelial ovarian cancer after adoptive transfer of tumor-infiltrating lymphocytes. Clinical Cancer Research. 1995. Available from: https://www.ncbi.nlm.nih.gov/pubmed/9816009

Chapter 2

The Role of Epigenetics in Cervical Cancer

Yair Alfaro-Mora, Luis A. Herrera,
Rodrigo Cáceres-Gutiérrez, Marco A. Andonegui-Elguera,
Guadalupe Dominguez-Gómez and José Díaz-Chávez

Abstract

Cervical cancer is the fourth most common type of cancer among women worldwide resulting in 528,475 new cases and 268,224 deaths. The principal etiological factor of cervical cancer is the persistent infection with high-risk types of human papillomaviruses (HPV), however is not sufficient, other factors like age, smoking, oral contraceptives, and genetic background are implicated in the development of this neoplasia. Although the understanding of cervical carcinogenesis has been increasing in recent decades, the epigenetic modifications (DNA methylation, histone modification, miRNAs and long non-coding RNAs) and its contribution to the development of cervical cancer remain largely unknown. In the next chapter, we will recapitulate the described findings on the alteration of epigenetic factors that, together with the persistent infection of HPV, could contribute to the malignant and invasive phenotype in cervical cancer.

Keywords: HPV, DNA methylation, histone modification, ncRNAs, therapy

1. Introduction

Cervical cancer is the fourth most common type of cancer among women worldwide, resulting in 528,475 new cases per year with 268,224 deaths [1]. Cervical cancer represents 6.6% of all female cancers and nearly 90% of all deaths occur in both low- and middle-income countries, as the disease is detected in the advanced stages or when the treatment is inaccessible [2]. The principal etiological factor of cervical cancer is the persistent infection with high-risk types of human papillomaviruses (hr-HPV). In fact, the HPV prevalence among women with normal cytology worldwide was 11.7%. This estimate varies by geography being Sahara African regions (24%), Latin America and the Caribbean (16.2%), Eastern Europe (14.2%), and Southeaster Asia (14%) the regions with the highest percentage of prevalence [3].

Most of hr-HPV premalignant lesions have a spontaneously viral clearance with a mean of 3 months in age-independent manner. Nonetheless, the cytological regression takes a longer time. This period depends in great manner on the grade of the lesion and if one or several hr-HPV are present. While mild and moderate/severe premalignant lesions with no HPV presence takes a mean of 5–6 months to recovery; mild, moderated, or severe premalignant lesions with the presence of hr-HPV takes a mean of 17, 24, and 60 months, respectively [4, 5]. However, although hr-HPV persistent infection is necessary for the development of cervical cancer, the solely infection is not sufficient. The presence of factors like age [6, 7], smoking [8], oral contraceptives [9], alcohol usage [10], and host and viral genetic background are necessary to observe an accumulation of epithelial cell abnormalities like sustained proliferation and growth of new blood vessels. These abnormalities emerge due to genomic alteration, defects in the genome maintenance and repair, destabilization of the number of DNA copies, and/or somatic mutations. Then, the cells that harbor all these abnormalities can evolve progressively to a tumorigenic, and further, a malignant and invasive phenotype [11].

2. Papillomaviruses

HPVs are DNA viruses that are able to infect the skin or mucosa of animal species. More than 200 human papillomavirus genotypes are known and have been categorized into phylogenetic genera as Alpha, Beta, Gamma, Mu, and Nu. The high-risk types of the Alpha genus are sexually transmitted being the types 16, 18, 52, 31, 58, 39, 51, and 56 the most common hr-HPV type found in women with apparent normal cytology. hr-HPV16 is the most frequently detected followed by hr-HPV18 and both are present in 70% of all the cervical cancers [12].

Papillomaviruses consist of a circular double-stranded DNA genome of approximately 8000 base pairs that harbor two main DNA structures: a long control region (LCR) which contains union sites for both, host cellular transcription factors and the viral proteins E1 and E2 that control viral replication and gene expression; and the open reading frames that codify to eight genes necessary for the maintenance and replication of the viral DNA. The high-risk alpha papillomaviruses present two well-characterized promoters: late promoter (LP or p670) which regulate gene expression of late proteins L1 and L2; and early promoter (PE or p97) which controls gene expression of early proteins E1, E2, E4, E5, E6, and E7. These genes are expressed by a complex pattern of mRNA splicing at different stages of the viral life cycle. The early and late viral proteins exert different function in the infected cell. E1 and E2 are involved in the viral genome replication, L1 and L2 orchestrate the virus assembly, and the E4, E5, E6, and E7 alter the replication machinery of the infected cell to facilitate the virus replication. Due to the target of the viral proteins E6 and E7 in the host cell, these proteins have been termed viral oncoproteins [13, 14].

The main interaction partner of HPV-E6 is the E3 ubiquitin ligase E6-asociated protein (E6AP) which in turn targets the tumor suppressor p53 and proteins with a PDZ domain to proteasomal degradation to promote de-differentiation, impairing apoptosis induction, and eliminate cell cycle checkpoints of the infected cell [15–17]. HPV-E7 binds to multiple proteins of the Rb family members, such as pRb, p107, and p130 (collectively referred as pocket proteins) that is more extensively studied. hr-HPV E7 uses a short stretch of residues known as LXCXE motif and residues in its N-terminus interact and target degradation of the three Rb family members. The proteasome-mediated destruction of E7/Rb pocket proteins is mediated by the recruitment of Cullin 2 E3 ubiquitin ligase complex, allowing the infected cell to remain in a proliferative state [18–20]. It has been observed that a correlation between viral DNA integration to host cell genomic material and a higher expression of E6 and E7 viral protein, provides an advantage in the cellular growing and oncogenic progression by promoting cell proliferation, abrogating the cell cycle checkpoints, and causes genomic instability [21–23]. Since HPV is considered the principal risk factor in cervical cancer, it is also associated with other cancer types like vulvar, vaginal, anal, penile, and oropharyngeal in females and males, the Advisory Committee on Immunization Practices (ACIP) recommend the routine vaccination with one of the three commercial available vaccines against HPV (9-valent, 4-valent, and 2-valent HPV vaccines, (HPVV)) in females and males at age 11 or 12 years and females aged 11–26 years and males aged 13 through 21 years not vaccinated previously. 2vHPVV contains HPV 16,18 virus-like particles; 4vHPVV contains HPV 6, 11, 16, and 18 virus-like particles; and 9vHPVV 6, 11, 16, 18, 31, 33, 45, 52, and 58 virus-like particles. These vaccines show a CIN prevention efficacy of 98% [24, 25]. Based in the above observations, these data highlight the importance of vaccination against HPVs since it seems like the expression of the HPV genome is the first step for development of pre-cancer lesions and a possible malignant progression. In this chapter, we review activities of E6 and E7 modulating epigenetics in cervical cancer and how these modifications could contribute to the development of this neoplasia.

Traditionally, cancer has been viewed as a multifactorial genetic disease that raise from an accumulation of mutations in tumor suppressor and/or oncogenes that cause loss or gain of function and an abnormal genetic expression. Although the understanding of cervical carcinogenesis has been increasing in recent decades, the epigenetic modifications (DNA methylation, histone modification and non-coding RNA (ncRNA)) and its contribution to the development of cervical cancer remain unknown. Nonetheless, in the past years, multiple epigenetic modifications have been associated with cancer initiation and proliferation [26]. The epigenetic are all the heritable changes in gene expression that are not due to changes in the nucleotide sequence of DNA. These modifications are established during embryonic development to bring cellular identity and are stably maintained during cellular replication in differentiated tissues. This is achieved by controlling the accessibility of transcription factors and by altering the capability of DNA packaging, having as result a temporal and spatial modulation in gene expression. Collectively, these modifications are referred as the epigenome. The epigenome comprises four main phenomena: Pos-translational histone modifications, DNA methylation, chromatin remodeling, and regulation by non-coding RNAs [26–28]. Recently, different works have been shown that hr-HPV E6 and E7 viral proteins have the capability of target key proteins which regulate epigenetic marks.

3. DNA methylation

The DNA methylation is associated with gene silencing due the recruitment and/or disassociation of DNA-binding proteins that can act as repressor complexes or transcription factors which generate a transcriptional silencing. Moreover, the methylation is necessary for a correct embryonic development [15], genome stability [16], X chromosome inactivation [17, 18], genomic imprinting [19], and silence of retrotransposons [20]. In mammals, the predominant form of DNA methylation occurs by a covalent addition of a methyl group in the fifth carbon of cytosine residues that are preceded by guanine nucleotides (CpG dinucleotides) in both DNA strands. This methyl group comes from a universal donor called S-adenosyl-L-methionine (SAM) and the enzymatic reaction is controlled by 3 DNA methyltransferases named DNMT1, DNMT3A, and DNMT3B, and the enzymatically inactive proteins DNMT2 and DNMT3L [21, 22]. Nearly 80% of all the DNA CpG dinucleotides in somatic tissues are methylated and comprises satellite DNAs, repetitive elements like transposons, non-repetitive intergenic DNA, and exons of genes [23]. From this DNA elements, there are CpG dinucleotides that are non-methylated that can be detected in germ cells, early embryo, and in somatic tissues.

These CpG dinucleotides are concentrated in short DNA stretches whit an overage length from 500 to 2000 base pairs (bp) that are known as CpG Islands (CGIs) [24]. The main characteristics of the CGIs are an elevated G + C base concentration, low CpG depletion, absence of DNA methylation, and are preferentially located at 5′end of genes, occupying approximately 60% of human gene promoters [25–27].

In general, DNA methylation of CpG around the Transcription Start Site (TSS) is negatively correlated with gene expression, whereas a low DNA methylation around TSS and a high DNA methylation in the gene body are positively correlated with gene expression [28]. It has been reported that DNMT3A is overexpressed in HPV positive tumors and that DNMT1 overexpression leads to an increased overall DNA methylation and transformation of NIH 3 T3 cells [29, 30]. Also, it has been shown an increase in DNMT1 protein levels in low-grade CIN and in SCC in comparison with normal epithelium [31]. These observations positioned DNMT1 as a regulator of tumor progression. Interestingly, the analysis of genome wide methylation in squamous carcinoma (SCC) cell lines reveals that in SCC cells HPV positive harbors higher CpG methylation in repetitive regions and in genic and non-genic non-repetitive regions in comparison to SCC HPV negative cells [30]. This HPV-mediated DNA methylation increase can be explained by the modulation of E6 and E7 proteins over the expression and activity of the DNA methylation machinery that is described as follow.

The DNMT1 is known as maintenance methyltransferase. During the DNA replication, DNMT1 ensures that hemi-methylated CpG sites in the newly synthesized DNA maintain the methylation patterns accurately using as template for parental strand [32], whereas Dnmt3A and Dnmt3b mediate the de novo DNA methylation and establish the pattern of methylation in embryonic development [33]. The DNMT1 gene expression is controlled by the complex conformed by the tumor suppressor p53, transcription factor Specificity Protein 1 (SP1), and the Histone Deacetylases 1 and 6 (p53-SP1-HDAC1/6). This complex binds to SP1 binding sites near the DNMT1 promoter [34]. When present, E6 oncoprotein collaborates to increase the DNMT1 expression. In vitro assays shown that HPV16-E6 increases DNA methylation levels by stimulating expression and activity of DNMT1 by p53 suppression [35, 36]. As p53 is targeted to degradation by hr-HPV-E6 and E3 ubiquitin ligase E6-asociated protein (E6AP) [37], the complex p53-SP1-HDAC1/6 could be disrupted increasing the levels of SP1 in the cell and leading to an SP1-mediated DNMT1 protein expression. Moreover, it has been shown that if SP1 protein levels increases, it is capable to target p53 to degradation by MDM2-mediated ubiquitination [34]. On the other hand, E7 oncoprotein binds directly to DNMT1 mediated by the C-terminal zinc-finger CR3 domain of E7, upregulating the methyltransferase activity and stabilizing the DNMT1 protein [38, 39]. This direct activation of DNMT1 by E7 could be potentiated in a positive feedback manner since the transcription of the gene is regulated by pRB/E2F1 [40]. Interestingly, Cicchini and colleagues shown that near E7-dependent hypermethylated clusters are an enrichment of EPAS1, FOXJ3, CDX2, IRF4, FOXF1, and GCR transcription factor binding motifs, suggesting that HPV16-E7 is capable to direct DNMT1 to silence gene promoters through an E7-transcription factor interaction [41]. Although it has been reported that the interaction of E7 with different transcription factors [42–44] and cells expressing hr-HPV viral DNA harbors a plethora of hypermethylated genes [30, 41, 45–54] (See **Table 1**), further experiments are needed to clarify this data.

The ability of HPV to maintain a persistent infection resides on mechanisms of immune host response evasion. The major histocompatibility complex (MHC-I) α-subunit HLA-E is significantly downregulated by hypermethylation in a distant regulatory CpG island by HPV16-E7 suggesting that E7 alters immune cell

Gene	Reference	Gene	Reference
APC	[55]	MGMT	[45, 48, 49]
C8ORF4	[56]	MRC2	[54]
C13ORF18	[51]	MT1G	[57]
CADM1	[50]	NKX2-8	[54]
CCNA1	[58, 59]	NMES1	[56]
CCND2	[60]	NPTX-1	[54]
CDH1	[46, 56, 61]	p16	[46, 48]
CDH13	[60]	P73	[62]
CDKN2A	[49]	PHACTR3	[54]
CLIC3	[54]	PRDM14	[54]
CNNA1	[51, 58, 59]	PTEN	[63]
CREB3LI	[54]	RAR-62	[64]
CxCL 14	[65]	RARB	[60]
DAPK	[45, 46, 49, 60]	RASSF1A	[66]
DDK3	[53]	RASSF2	[52]
E-cadherin	[67]	RRAD	[56]
H-cadherin	[67]	SFRP1	[56]
EPB41L3	[52]	SFRP2	[53]
FAM19A4	[54]	SFRP4	[53]
FHIT	[47, 49]	SFRP5	[53]
HLA-E	[41]	SLCA4	[54]
FLJ36166	[56]	SOST	[54]
FN1	[56]	SOX17	[53]
GPNMB	[56]	SPARC	[56]
HSPA2	[56]	SSX4	[56]
hTERT	[45, 48, 49, 51]	TFPI2	[56]
INK4A	[48]	TIMP-3	[46]
LFNG	[54]	TNFSF13	[54]
LHX1	[54]	TSCL1	[68]
MAL	[50]	TWIST1	[51, 60]
		WDFY3	[54]

Table 1.
Cervical cancer genes hypermethylated reported in literature.

recognition during early stages of persistent infection [41]. On the other hand, CxCL 14 is a chemokine that functions as a potent angiogenesis inhibitor and a chemotactic factor for dendritic and natural killer cells [69, 70]. It has been seen that E7 downregulates the chemokine CXCL14 by a direct hypermethylation of its promoter. If the CxCL14 expression is restored, an increase of the presence of natural killer and CD8+ T cells in tumor-draining lymph nodes is observed [65]. HPV also inhibit the ability of Langerhans cells (antigen presenting cells) to infiltrate into the virus infected area by reducing the E-cadherin expression on infected keratinocytes cell membrane [71]. It has been demonstrated that in oral tongue, breast, and prostate cell lines as well as breast and prostate tumors that Enhancer of Zeste Homolog 2 (EZH2), Embryonic Ectoderm Development (EED), and Suppressor of Zeste 12 (ZUS12), components of the Polycomb Repressive Complex 2 (PCR2) along with Histone Deacetylase 1 (HDAC1) are responsible of E-cadherin silencing by Histone 3 lysine 27 trimethylation (H3K27me3) on E-cadherin promoter [72, 73]. Since it has been reported that HPV16-E6 and E7 induce a decrease in the transcription levels of E-cadherin gene without targeting E-cadherin to proteasome degradation or methylation of the E-cadherin promoter [36, 39], this PRC2 silencing mechanism could be the responsible of E7-mediated E-cadherin-downregulation due E7 can induce EZH2 expression via liberation of E2F transcription factors from the inhibitory activity of pRB, p107, and p130 [74]. EZH2 increase expression could arise the formation of PRC2 that, in turn, can recruit and hyperactivate type 1 Histone Deacetylases (HDAC-1) leading to histone deacetylation and a subsequent trimethylation in H3K27 at the E-cadherin promoter silencing its expression [75, 76]. In addition, it has been shown that hr-HPV16 E7 can block HDAC-HIF-1α interaction [77] leading to a possible increase in HDAC free levels that can interact with PCR2. Moreover, HPV16/18 E6 and E7 oncoproteins increase the expression of thymopoietin pseudogene 2 (TMPOP2; lncRNA-EBIC) a long non-coding RNA that is repressed in cis by p53 transcription factor (see below). This lncRNA-EBIC can interact with EZH2 generating a TMPOP2-EZH2 complex that has been postulated as a PRC2-recruit facilitator to E-cadherin promoter region silencing these gene [78, 79].

Although the hypermethylation gene status is predominant in the hr-HPV host cell genome, there are works that demonstrate a hypomethylation in promotor genes (See **Table 2**). Yin et al., analyzed the expression and promoter methylation status of STK31 gene in cell lines and cervical tumors expressing hr-HPV. They found an increased expression and a hypomethylation of STK31 CpG islands in HPV16/18-positive HeLa, SiHa, and CaSki cervical cancer cell lines and HPV16/18-positive pre-malignant lesion Cervical Intraepithelial Neoplasia grade 3 (CIN3) and Cervical Cancer (CC) biopsies compared with HPV-negative C33A and HT-3 cervical cancer cell lines and HPV-negative CIN3 and CC. In addition, the authors reported that STK31 promotor were hypermethylated in all normal, CIN1, and CIN2 biopsies analyzed. However, STK3 promoter were hypomethylated in all CIN3 and CC biopsies analyzed being found more often hypomethylated in CIN3 than in CC [82]. Other genes found to be hypomethylated were Rap guanidine Nucleotide Exchange Factor (RAPGEF1) and Cancer Antigen Gene (CAGE). Samuelsson and colleagues shown that 48% of cervical squamous carcinomas analyzed present no methylation in CGI near RAPGEF1 promoter and hypomethylation on a CGI present in the first intron of these gene [80]. Lee and colleagues analyzed the methylation status of CAGE promotor gene in 40 cervical cancer patients finding that 87.5% of the samples where hypomethylated in comparison of control non-neoplastic tissues [81].

Gene	Reference
RAPGEF1	[80]
CAGE	[81]
STK31	[82]
COL17A1	[83]
Ribosomal DNA	[84]

Table 2.
Cervical cancer genes hypomethylated reported in literature.

Interestingly, HPV16 DNA is an efficient target for DNA methylation by host cell DNA methylation machinery. The viral DNA is organized into nucleosomes in equal form that eukaryote DNA [85, 86]. This viral DNA organization can modulate the viral gene expression by DNA methylation and histone modifications. The E2 viral protein is the master regulator of E6 and E7 expression by binding into four conserved E2-binding sites (E2BS) that are located in the LCR close to DNA binding sites of several cellular transcription factors like TATA-binding protein, AP-1, Sp1, GPS2/AMF-1, TopoBP1, CDP, and YY1. These E2BS have a consensus DNA sequence 5′-ACCG(n)4CGGT-3′ upstream of the p97 early promoter. The E2 viral protein can activate or repress viral transcription in a dose dependent manner. At low concentrations E2 binds to E2BS4 due its great affinity, leaving the E6 promoter active. When E2 rises, the low affinity binding sites E2BS1 and E2BS2 are occupied by E2 blocking the binding of transcription factors and the recruitment of transcriptional repressors at the E6 promoter, preventing E6 and E7 transcription [87–91]. In addition, E2 is able to bind the double bromodomain protein Brd4, through of its C-terminal region and the bromodomain-containing region BDR4 recruits E2 viral protein by its N-terminal and C-terminal DNA binding domain region to E2BS-4, thus preventing the Transcription Factor II D (TFIID) and polymerase II interaction with TATA box and E6 promotor region, respectively [92]. The E2-BDR4 complex also represses the interaction between BDR4 and the Positive Transcription Elongation Factor b (P-TEFb) which is necessary to E6 and E7 expression [93]. In this way, the loss of regulation of the E2 viral protein deregulate the expression of E6 and E7 viral proteins, which can in turn contribute to further malignant transformation. HPV genome integration usually occurs in the E1 and E2 ORF regions generating a loss of E2 negative expression control allowing unregulated transcription of E6 and E7 viral genes [90, 94]. The viral integration has been shown to occur in two different ways: as a single genome and a head-to-tail multiple tandem repeats correlating positively the amount of CpG methylation with the number of integrated viral genome copies [95–97]. If multiple viral DNA copies are integrated in host genome, only one copy is transcriptionally active due a extensively methylation of the other integrated genome viral copies [95]. Otherwise, has been shown in vitro that E2 viral protein E2BSs binding capability is impaired by CpG methylation being more prevalent E2BS1 site methylated. These E2BSs methylation in the HPV16 LCR trigger the overexpression of E6 and E7 viral proteins [95, 97–99]. Moreover, the grade of methylation in E2BSs and in LCR varies in great manner depending of the differentiated status of the host cell, being highly methylated in less well differentiated cells and hypomethylated in LCR of viral genomes in more highly differentiated epithelial cells, correlating with the E6 and E7 course expression in infecting cells [100]. In addition to disruption of E2 ORF, the methylation of specific CpG present in hr-HPV LCR leads to an increase expression of E6 and E7 viral genes even if E2 viral protein still expressing in the host cell. All these observations underscore the combined mechanisms conducted by E6 and E7 in the methylation and hypomethylation to achieve an optimum environment for viral replication.

4. Pos-translational histone modifications

It is importantly to note that the E6 and E7 capability of altering gene expression can occur by interaction with a subset of chromatin-modifying enzymes that are flanking target genes. In higher eukaryotes and double-stranded DNA viruses, the DNA is tightly wrapping around a heterogeneous multi-unit structure termed nucleosome. The nucleosome is the core unit of chromatin which is 146-bp length

DNA wound around octameric of the four highly conserved histone proteins (H3, H4, H2A, and H2B). Each nucleosome is linked one to other by a stretch of DNA called DNA linker with a length of 40–55 bp. The chromatin gives DNA structure and regulates the gene transcription via post-translational modifications (PTM). This PTM are modifications such acetylation, methylation, phosphorylation, ubiquitination, sumoylation, glycosylation, homocysteinylation, crotonylation, propionylation, and butyrylation in the amino-terminal and carboxy-terminal tail of histones that are mediated by diverse histone modifying enzymes. These PTM regulate gene expression by affecting the nucleosome stability and structure [101, 102].

The E6 and E7 viral proteins can alter the chromatin structure by association and/or modifying the enzymatic activity and/or altering the expression of chromatin-remodeling enzymes. HPV16-E7 modulates the immune host response downregulating a subset of proteins by methylation. Viral nucleic acids are sensed by a pathogen recognition receptor (PRR) called toll-like receptor 9 (TLR9) that are expressed in keratinocytes. This receptor allows the recognition of unmethylated double-stranded DNA CpG motifs present in the HPV DNA and initiate a signaling cascade that leads to the production of type I Interferon (INF) and proinflammatory cytokines which in turn activates host immune defenses against the infection. Nonetheless, in vitro experiments have been shown that HPV16-E7 suppress TLR9 transcription by inducing the formation of a repressive chromatin modification complex witch is formed by ERα, HDAC1, JARID1B, and NF-kB p50-p65 at specific NF-kB element (site B) of TLR9 promoter. Recruited by ERα, JARID1B prevents the trimethylation of histone 3 at lysin 4 (H3K4me3) and HDAC-1 prevents the acetylation of histone 4 (AcH4) from the site B until the transcription start site of the TLR9 promoter in C33A cells with HPV16 [103]. However, two different reports observed that TLR9 expression was only expressed in fully differentiated keratinocytes and in different layers of HPV-positive cervical epithelia neoplasia and that TLR9 expression is primary intracellular in cervical epithelium [104, 105]. Another study conducted by Canella and collaborators observed that TLR9 expression under presence of low-risk or high-risk HPV and an increase in the TLR9 protein expression in patients with persistent HPV infection. The authors argue that the discrepancies in the TLR9 expression in HPV infected cells reside in a balance between the strength of TLR9 inhibition by HPV and the subject capability to drive proper TLR9 activation [106]. However, further studies are needed to elucidate this data discrepancy.

HPV16-E7 also interferes with downstream signaling of TLRs. It has been seen that E7 interacts in vivo and in vitro with the Interferon Regulatory Factor-1 (IRF-1). IRF-1 is a transcription factor how belong to a family of 9 DNA-binding factors are called from IRF-1 to IRF-9. IRF-1 recognizes a central 11–13 nucleotide core region denominated INF stimulated response elements (ISREs) [107]. These regulatory elements are present in the promoters of INF-β and some INF-inducible genes [108]. HPV16-E7 interacts directly with its CR1/2 domains and the carboxyl-terminal transactivation domain of IRF-1, eliminating its transactivation function of IRF-1 both in vitro and in vivo. Moreover, the Nucleosome remodeling and deacetylase (NuRD) complex could be implicated since HPV16-E7 interacts directly with Mi2β (a subunit of the NuRD complex) via C-terminal zinc-finger CR3 domain leading to a chromatin deacetylation and silencing IRF-1-dependent transcription suppressing cellular immune response due viral infection [109, 110].

E6 and E7 viral proteins can alter the activity of histone acetyltransferases (HAT) and histone deacetylases (HDAC). NF-κB is a transcription factor composed of homodimers or heterodimers complexes of five subunits named p50, p52, p65/Rel A, c-Rel, and Rel B; being p50/p65 the most common dimmer. To achieve a correct NF-κB transcription, it is necessary the recruitment and interaction with different transcriptional coactivators like CREB binding protein (CBP), p300, Steroid Receptor-Coactivator-1 (SRC-1), or Nuclear receptor CoAtivator-1 (NCoA-1) [111]. This interaction is mediated by Protein Kinase A (PKA) phosphorylation in p65/Rel A serine 276 residue unmasking the CPB-interaction domain present in p65/Rel A. This phosphorylation generates a conformational change that permits a bivalent interaction; first with CBP KIX domain (450–679 aa) and 276 phosphorylated p65-serine and last with CBP region comprised by 313–450 aa CBP and p65 region flanked by 477–504 aa [112]. The transcription of multiple p53-regulated genes is mediated by cyclic-AMP-regulated enhancer (CRE) transcription factor (CREB) and the HAT CBP, p300, and HMT PRMT1, CARM1, and SET7 coactivators that modulate the methylation and acetylation of histones surrounding p53 target genes [113, 114]. The complex CREB–CBP can bind to specific transcription factors where recruit and bind with histone binding factor RbAp48. This CREB–CBP-RbAp48 complex allows the interaction and subsequent CBP/p300 acetylation of target genes histones leading to a chromatin structure rearrange and recruitment of transcription machinery [115–120]. Moreover, An and coworkers demonstrated that in vivo and in vitro PRMT1 and CARM1 interacts directly with p53 trough N-terminal (1–43 aa) and C-terminal (370–393 aa), respectively. Also, they shown that are a cooperatively functions in p53 transcription by p300, PRMT1, and CARM1 coactivators for an optimal p53 transcription activity, being necessary the ordered recruitment to p53-responsive genes: first PRMT1 is recruited and methylate H4R3, then a p300 accumulation and H4 acetylation, and last a subsequent CARM1 accumulation and H3R17 methylation [114]. Like phosphorylation, it has been shown in vitro and in vivo that p53 can be activated and stabilized against ubiquitin-mediated degradation by SET7-mediated mono-methylation in residue 372 (p53-K372me1) and, presumably, a subsequent CBP/p300-mediated acetylation [121, 122]. The CBP/p300-p53 complex can interact with multiple p300 and p53 domains. It has been shown that p300 domains like N-terminal Taz1 domain (CH1 domain; 302–451 aa), KIX domain (588–683 aa), C-terminal Taz2 domain (CH3 domain; 1514–1737 aa), and nuclear receptor coactivator binding domain (NCBD; 2059–2117 aa) can interact with p53 TAD (1–61 aa) and DNA-binding Core Domain (90–160 aa) [123–127]. This CBP/p300-p53 interaction promotes p53 C-terminal domain (363–393 aa) acetylation leading to increase in p53-DNA binding and transcription activity in vivo and in vitro [123, 124, 128, 129].

Lee and coworkers demonstrated that p53 TAD multisite phosphorylation enhances p53 affinity for Taz1, Taz2, and KIX domains of CBP leading to a graded p53 response to genotoxic stress [130]. On other side, in vivo and in vitro experiments shown that the second zinc finger present in C-terminal region of HPV 16/18-E6 (aa 100–107) interact with CBP/p300 via its Transcriptional Adapter Motif (TRAM), a 19-aa sequence present in CBP II domain, competing with the CBP/p300-p53 interaction [131]. Also, has been shown that E6 interacts with p300 CH1 domain (340–413 aa) and NCBD domain (1970–2220 aa) generating a E6-p53-p300 complex without E6AP participation. This trimeric complex inhibits both p300-mediated acetylation of p53 and nucleosomal core histones abrogating the p53-dependent transcription activated by CBP/p300. In addition to a p53-E6-E6AP, in vitro and in vivo, HPV18-E6 promotes p53 degradation by direct association and inhibition of SET7 methyltransferase activity that stabilizes p53 by mono-methylation in K372 residue. Whereas not all p53 is promoted to degradation due loss of K372me1, HPV18-E6 can abolishes the p53-dependent remnant gene transcription by direct interaction and downregulation of coactivators CARM1, PRMT1, and SET7 methyltransferase activities, generating a reduced p53 DNA binding and loss of p53 gene expression [122]. Notably, DNMT1 is associated and monomethylated in K142 residue (DNMT1-K142) by SET7 causing its degradation [132]. Thus, it is possible that the presence of E6 abrogates the SET7-dependent degradation of DNMT1 increasing the free protein levels that can interact with E7 viral protein, generating an increased activity earlier described of DNMT1-E7 protein complex. Further experiments needed to demonstrate this hypothesis.

Also, hr-HPV 16-E6 disrupt the NF-κB-dependent transactivation by binding competition on N-terminus CH1 domain and C-terminus of CBP that are recognition sites of RelA/p65 and SCR-1, respectively. Furthermore, HPV16-E7 also suppresses the NF-κB-dependent transactivation. The N terminal (1–51 aa) region of E7 viral protein interact both in vitro and in vivo with TAZ2 domain of transcriptional coactivator CBP/p300. Notably, this interaction increases if HPV16-E7 CKII site (Ser31 and Ser32) is phosphorylated [129, 133–137]. hr-HPV16-E7 also can bind to P/CAF HAT domain (352–658 aa) via E7-leucine 67 residue diminishing P/CAF acetyltransferase activity [135].

5. HPV RNA targets

It has been described that, in humans, less than 3% of genome encodes to protein-coding exons while more than 85% of genome is transcribed into non-coding RNAs (ncRNAs) [138, 139]. These ncRNAs can be classified accordingly by their size as short or long ncRNAs. Micro RNAs (miRNAs) are a group of small non-coding single-strand RNA of 19–24 nucleotides that play key roles in differentiation and development by post-transcriptional regulation of cellular genes. Their main function is to repress the expression of target mRNA by cleavage or translational silencing depending of the degree of miRNA sequence complementation with the 3′-UTR of target mRNAs [140]. The HPV viral proteins can target different RNA species modifying their expression (See **Tables 3–5**). For example, HPV16 E2 and E6 viral proteins interact with RNA molecules and reduce the pre-RNA splice efficiency. The N-terminal trans activation domain and the hinge region of HPV16-E2 (1–220 aa and 221–259 aa respectively) and the central region of HPV16-E6 (42–102 aa) are the responsibly of splicing suppression; whereas the E2 C-terminal DNA-binding domain (260–365 aa) and the E6 C-terminal Nuclear Localization Signal (NLS3) domain (115–124 aa) are the protein portions responsible for protein-RNA interaction. Moreover, HPV16-E2 can interact with splicing factors SRp30, SRp40, SRp55, and SRp75 and HPV16-E6 interacts with SRp30, SRp55, and SRp75 via C-terminal of both viral proteins [173]. miRNA-23b is located in the intron 14 of the host gene C9ORF3 on chromosome 9. This miRNA regulates c-MET gene which mediates cellular apoptosis via AKT signaling pathway. When HPV16-E6 is present, C9ORF3 and the intronic miRNA-23b is downregulated by DNMT1-mediated CGI hypermethylation located 1 kb upstream from the transcription start site of C9ORF3 gene [174].

The miR-375 has been shown to regulate the HPV viral gene expression in vitro and in vivo. miR-375 can downregulates E6 and E7 viral transcription due the presence of two putative binding sites present in the E7 region (677–698 aa; 687–708 aa) and three in the E1 region (1236–1258 aa; 1259–1280 aa; 1862–1884 aa) of the HPV genome. Also, this miRNA in vivo and in vitro can bind directly the 3′UTR of E6AP and the transcription factor SP1 diminishing E6AP and SP1 mRNA and protein. As a result of E6AP and SP1 proteins degradation mediated by miR-375, an increase in p21, p53, and Rb proteins can be observed [175–177]. However, in vitro assays demonstrated that HPV16-E6 can hypermethylate DNMT1-mediated miR-375 promoter region [178] downregulating miR-375 and leading an increase in SP1 transcription factor levels, thereby, contributing to DNMT1-positive loop feedback

Gene up-regulated	Reference	Gene down-regulated	*Reference*
AC007879.7	[144]	MEG3	[153,154]
CCAT	[160, 161]	MIR205HG	[144]
CCEPR	[163]	OIS1	[155]
CCHE1	[142, 143]	PVT1	[156]
FAM83H	[144]	RP3-510D11.2	[144]
GAS5	[144]	RP6-65G23.3	[144]
GS1-600G8.5	[144]	RP11-479G22.8	[144]
H19	[144]	RP13.463N16.6	[144]
HOTAIR	[149]	RSU1P2	[157]
HOXC-As5	[144]	SFTA1P	[144]
LINC00963	[144]	SNHG15	[144]
LINC01057	[144]	SPRY4-IT1	[159]
lncRNA LET	[151]	TMPOP2 (lncRNA-EBIC)	[79]
MAFG-AS1	[144]	XIST	[162]
MALAT1	[152]	XLOC_010588	[164]

Table 3.
lncRNAs reported up- and down-regulated in literature.

described early. Moreover, miR-124 and miR-375 mediated a reciprocal regulation with long non-coding RNA MALAT1. If miR-375 is overexpressed a significant reduction in MALAT1 expression is observed. This regulation could be by direct interaction between miR-375 and MALAT1 due miR-375 has two putative MALAT1 binding sites whereas MALAT1 harbors two putative binding sites with miR-124 [169, 178]. Future experiments are necessary to elucidate which factors influence the downregulation of both, cellular and viral gene expression and the molecular factors are involved in HPV E6 and E7 interaction with these miRNAs and MALAT1.

Otherwise, the long non-coding RNAs (lncRNAs) are transcripts of more than 200 nucleotides in length. These RNAs possess structural characteristics of messenger RNAs (mRNAs) like that are transcribed by RNA Polymerase II, spliced, harbor a poly adenylated tail, and a 5′-caping. lncRNAs can modulate transcription, alternative splicing, mRNA stability, mRNA translation and chromatin remodeling by bind to RNA, DNA, or a subset of proteins. Interestingly, Khalil and colleagues showed that the mammalian genome encodes nearly 4500 lncRNAs and approximately 24% of these lncRNAS interact with chromatin-modifying proteins like the repressive complex PRC2, CoREST, and SCMX [179]. Due their role in distinct cellular processes, HPV viral proteins can modulate multiple host's lncRNAs [140].

As described earlier, the long non-coding RNA metastasis-associated lung adenocarcinoma transcript 1 (MALAT1) was associated with cell proliferation and invasion in HPV positive cervical cancer cells [152, 169, 180]. Also, in CaSki cell line, the transfection of MALAT1 increases the expression of cyclin D1, cyclin E and cyclin-dependent kinase 6 (CDK6). When HPV16 E6 and E7 are downregulated, MALAT1 expression is downregulated too, indicating that these viral proteins are involved in the MALAT1 expression [152]. However, further studies are needed to elucidate the mechanism of MALAT1 regulation by HPV.

Barr and colleagues identify a subset of lncRNAs upper and downregulated in primary human foreskin keratinocytes which express HPV16-E6 viral protein. The

Gene up-regulated	Reference	Gene up-regulated	Reference	Gene up-regulated	Reference
let-7e	[165]	miR-181c	[165, 172]	miR-30b	[165]
let-7i	[165]	miR-182	[170]	miR-30d	[165]
miR-106a	[167, 168]	miR-183	[170]	miR-30e	[165]
miR-106b	[168, 171, 172]	miR-185	[168]	miR-326	[165]
miR-10	[165]	miR-186	[165]	miR-339-5p	[168]
miR-10b	[168]	miR-187	[165]	miR-340	[165]
miR-1224-5p	[168]	miR-192	[172]	miR-342	[165]
miR-124	[172]	miR-194	[165]	miR-34a	[165]
miR-126	[165]	miR-195	[165]	miR-34c	[165]
miR-127	[165]	miR-196a	[141]	miR-374	[165]
miR-129	[165]	miR-199a	[165]	miR-449a	[172]
miR-130a	[165]	miR-199b	[165]	miR-449b	[172]
miR-130b	[165, 168]	miR-199s	[165]	miR-512-3p	[172]
miR-132	[141, 165]	miR-19a	[165]	miR-517a	[172]
miR-133a	[165]	miR-20	[165]	miR-517c	[172]
miR-133b	[165]	miR-200a	[165]	miR-518f	[172]
miR-134	[165]	miR-200c	[170]	miR-542-3p	[172]
miR-135a	[165]	miR-205	[170]	miR-545	[172]
miR-135b	[165, 172]	miR-20a	[158, 167]	miR-625	[168]
miR-139	[165]	miR-20b	[168]	miR-7g	[165]
miR-140	[165]	miR-21	[145, 165, 168, 171]	miR-886-5p	[167]
miR-141	[172]	miR-210	[170]	miR-9	[165]
miR-142-3p	[165]	miR-213	[165]	miR-92a	[167]
miR-142-5p	[165]	miR-214	[165]	miR-93	[167, 168]
miR-145	[165]	miR-215	[165]	miR-941	[168]
miR-146	[165]	miR-218	[165]	miR-98	[165]
miR-146a	[166]	miR-223	[166]		
miR-146b-5p	[168]	miR-224	[167]		
miR-148a	[141]	miR-25	[165]		
miR-150	[165]	miR-26a	[165]		
miR-151	[165]	miR-26b	[165]		
miR-155	[166–168]	miR-28	[165]		
miR-15	[165, 166, 168]	miR-29a	[165]		
miR-15b	[166, 167, 171]	miR-29b	[165]		
miR-16	[167, 171, 172]	miR-301	[165]		
miR-17	[168]	miR-301b	[172]		
miR-181a	[165]	miR-302b	[141]		
miR-181b	[165]	miR-30a-3p	[165]		

Table 4.
miRNAs reported up-regulated in literature.

authors found that FAM83H-AS1 is overexpressed by HPV16-E6 viral protein mediated by p300, and its inhibition decrease proliferation, migration, and resistance to apoptosis in vitro, whereas in pre-malignant and cervical cancer tissues the

Gene	Reference	Gene	Reference
let-7a-c	[145]	miR-218	[99, 166, 167]
let-7b	[145]	miR-23b	[145, 166]
let-7c	[145]	miR-26a	[141]
miR-100	[168]	miR-29a	[167]
miR-101	[166]	miR-328	[168]
miR-10b	[167]	miR-34a	[166]
miR-124	[169]	miR-368	[170]
miR-125b	[167, 168, 171]	miR-370	[171]
miR-126	[167, 170]	miR-375	[167, 168]
miR-139-3p	[168]	miR-379	[168]
miR-139-5p	[168]	miR-381	[168]
miR-143	[166, 170]	miR-424	[166, 167]
miR-145	[166, 168, 170]	miR-433	[172]
miR-149	[168]	miR-494	[171]
miR-188	[171]	miR-497	[168, 170]
miR-193b	[171]	miR-513	[141]
miR-195	[167, 168, 170]	miR-572	[171]
miR-196b	[145]	miR-574-3p	[168]
miR-199a	[141]	miR-575	[171]
miR-199a-5p	[168]	miR-617	[168]
miR-199b-5p	[168]	miR-638	[171]
miR-203	[171]	miR-99a	[167, 168]

Table 5.
miRNAs reported down-regulated in literature.

high expression of FAM83H-AS1 correlates with worse overall survival compared with normal cervix samples [144].

The lncRNA HOX Transcript Antisense Intergenic RNA (HOTAIR) can binds to and recruits the PRC2 to repress transcription of multiple gene loci in trans. HOTAIR expression is downregulated in earlier stages of cervical cancer. However, in HPV16 positive cervical carcinomas and in HPV positive cell lines which harbor a higher HPV16-E7 protein expression, the lncRNA HOTAIR is upregulated correlating with high HPV16-E7 expression level. Moreover, HPV16-E7 interacts with HOTAIR. This interaction could impair the formation of the PCR2 complex generating diminish of H3K27me3 repression mark and thus increasing the expression of a large number of genes [149, 181, 182]. Interestingly, the HPV16-E7-HOTAIR interaction generates an autoregulatory loop between HOTAIR, miR-331-3p and Neuropilin 2 (NRP2). It has been shown that HOTAIR is a competitive endogenous RNA (ceRNA) showing a sponge effect over miR-331-3p and that miR-331-3p directly regulates NRP2. So, when is present, HPV16-E7 interacts and diminishes HOTAIR expression generating an increase of miR-331-3p levels due the lack of HOTAIR sponge effect over miR-331-3p. The miR-331-3p induce a decrease of NRP2 levels by binding through 3'UTR of NRP. Being NRP2 a HPV16-E7 transcription regulator, the downregulation of NRP2 protein levels lead to a diminished HPV16-E7 protein levels too, generating a regulatory loop [183, 184].

As described early, thymopoietin pseudogene 2 (TMPOP2, lncRNA-EBIC) is a lncRNA that interact with EZH2 to repress E-cadherin gene expression. Interestingly, this lncRNA regulates the expression of HPV viral genes in cervical cancer cells. Several miRNAs, like miR-375 and miR-139, can target to degradation the HPV16/18 E6 and E7 mRNA. However, lncRNA-EBIC also acts as a ceRNA, sequestering miR-375 and miR-139 increasing the E6 and E7 viral gene expression. Moreover, the upregulation of E6 and E7 by lncRNA-EBIC lead to p53 degradation which is a transcriptional repressor of lncRNA-EBIC, generating a positive loop feedback [79].

The lncRNA LET [151], GAS5 [146], and MEG3 [153, 154] expression is downregulated in cervical cancer tissues and is associated with poor prognosis, malignant status, lymph node metastasis, invasion, and shorter overall survival. The expression of MEG3 leads to an increase in cell apoptosis, increased levels of p53 and cleaved caspase 3 in cervical cancer cells. Also, this lncRNA can regulate the expression levels of miR-21-5p [153, 154].

On the contrary, the lnc Ras Suppressor Protein 1 Pseudogene 2 (RSU1P2) expression is upregulated in cervical cancer tissues and promotes proliferation, invasion, and migration of cervical cancer cell lines. Moreover, in vitro and in vivo assays demonstrated that RSU1P2 acts as ceRNA binding directly to and downregulating let7a expression, leading to an increase of Let-7a target genes as IGF1R, N-myc, and EphA4. Interestingly, let-7a can target the 3-UTR of N-Myc inhibiting its mRNA and protein production, whereas N-Myc can bind to RSU1P2 promoter region and increase its transcription. Therefore, N-Myc can forms a positive loop feedback with RSU1P2 increasing its oncogenic activity [157]. If any HPV viral protein can modulate this pathway is currently unknown.

The lncRNA Plasmacytoma Variant Translocation 1 (PVT1) expression is upregulated in cervical cancer tissues and correlates positively with poor overall survival. If PVT1 expression is inhibit a decrease in cellular proliferation, migration, and invasion is observed whereas apoptosis and cisplatin toxicity increase in cervical cancer cell lines [156].

There are numerous lncRNAs that have been poorly investigated in their molecular mechanism in HPV-infected cervical carcinoma cells. However, some studies described the correlations between lncRNAS expression and clinical characteristics of cervical cancer patients. For example, the lncRNA Colon Cancer-Associated Transcript 2 (CCAT2) [160, 161], SPRY4-IT1 [159], and CCHE1 [142] are highly expressed and positively associated with cell proliferation and survival of cervical cancer cells as well malignant status and poor prognosis of cervical cancer patients. CCHE1 high expression promotes cell proliferation of cervical cancer cells. Interestingly, CCHE1 physically interacts with Proliferating Cell Nuclear Antigen (PCNA) mRNA increasing the PCNA gene expression. This PCNA expression is necessary for the proliferation effect of CCHE1 [143].

6. Therapeutic approaches

The balance alteration of oncogenes and tumor-suppressor genes creates an advantage to cancer cells. Many of these alterations are due epigenetic alterations such DNA methylation, histone modification, and/or non-coding RNAs expression/repression. However, this cancer cells advantage can serve also as therapeutic targets to counterattack cancer pathogenesis and progression. Currently, there are some studies describing drugs that alter these epigenetic changes present in cervical cancer cells.

A study employs a peripheral vasodilator drug and DNA methylation inhibitor called Hydralazine. The authors employed hydralazine at 40 μmol/L for 72 h and they observed a restoration of APC gene expression in HeLa and CaSki cervical cancer cells. This gene re-expression was due to APC promoter region demethylation [55]. In 2005, Zambrano and colleagues mounted a phase 1 study of hydralazine employing different dosages (from 25 mg/8 h to 50 mg/8 h) for a 10 days period. They found that employing any hydralazine concentration tested, eight tumor suppressors genes were demethylate and re-expressed in untreated cervical cancer patients without affecting global DNA methylation [185].

Another compound capable to restore gene expression of tumor suppressor genes hypermethylated is Trichosanthin (TCS). TCS is a 237 aa type I ribosome-inactivating protein extracted from the root tubers of the Chinese medical herb *Trichocanthes kirilowi*. Huang and colleagues reported increases mRNA and protein levels of APC and TSLC1 due demethylation in the CpG islands in the promoter region in HeLa and CaSki cervical cancer cells treated with 20, 40 and 80 μg/ml for 48 h presumable mediated by DNMT1 since its mRNA, protein levels, and enzyme activity decreases following the treatment in a dose-dependent manner [68]. However, until these data shown a likely useful as a demethylating agent for treatment, this work does not report the toxicity effects over non-transformed cell lines.

In another study, hydralazine was proved in combination with the HDAC inhibitor valproate acid. After 5 days of Hydralazine at 10 μM and magnesium Valproate at 1 mM treatment, SiHa, CasKi, and HeLa cervical cancer cells lead to a small increase HPV gene expression due demethylation and acetylated H4 enrichment at 5'region of LCR. However, a p53 gene expression and protein levels were increased after treatment whit Hydralazine, Valproate, or in combination in CasKi, HeLa, and SiHa cell lines being p53 stability likely due 373 and 382 lysine p53 hyperacetylation that protects from E6-mediated degradation. Also, the hydralazine/valproate phase II trial with treatment of Hydralazine at 182 or 83 mg and magnesium Valproate at 40 mg/kg shown that E6 and E7 transcripts remains unchanged in primary tumors of patients with cervical cancer, suggesting that epigenetic therapy cannot facilitate increase of viral oncogene activation [186].

On the other hand, apicidin, an inhibitor of histone deacetylases, induces downregulation of DNMT1 and increase p21WAF1/Cip1 expression in HeLa cervical cancer cell line. The Apicidin-mediated DNMT1 downregulation is achieved by a significant H3 and H4 hypoacetylation, depletion of H3K4me3 gene transcription mark, and enriched H3K9me3 and H3K27me3 repressive marks in the nucleosomes on DNMT1 transcriptional initiation site. Moreover, Apicidin treatment lead to a decreased Pol II presence on the transcription initiation site and the recruitment of co-repressors pRB and HDAC1 and dissociation of activators P/CAF and HAT from the E2F consensus-binding site on the DNMT1 promoter site. However, HeLa cells treated solely with Apicidin does not induce apoptosis of HeLa cells in comparison of DNMT1 knock down which cause an apoptotic effect, indicating that other targets are needed to achieve Apicidin therapeutic effect [187].

Quercetin a flavonoid found in fruits and vegetables also have epigenetics effects, it has been reported that quercetin induces attenuating lipid peroxidation, platelet aggregation, capillary permeability, anti-proliferative, anti-migratory, and proapoptotic effect in HeLa cervical carcinoma cells [188]. Employing doses of 25 and 50 μM, Quercetin can inhibit the activity of DNMT1, HDACs, H3K9 HMT activity, in a dose-dependent manner. Using the same Quercetin concentrations was observed a decreased methylation percentage and increase APC, CDH1, CDH13, DAPK1, FHTI, GSTP1, MGMT, MLH1, PTEN, RARB, RASSF1, SOC51, TIMP3, and VHL expression and a global DNA methylation in a dose-dependent manner. Also, Quercetin modulates the expression of several enzymes and chromatin modifiers like HDAC2, HDAC1, DNMT1, HDAC3, HAT1, DNMT3B, HDAC7, HDAC6, HDAC11, DNMT3A, and HDAC5 in a dose-dependent manner [189]. Interestingly, those therapeutic approaches described here where tested employing cervical cancer models. However, it would be interesting explore the effectiveness of these approaches on HPV-infected anus and oral models where HPV is associated with malignant transformation [150, 190–192].

7. Conclusions

Here we describe the epigenetic regulation mechanisms observed when hr-HPV is present in cervical cancer. The viral oncoproteins expression from hr-HPV induce genetic and epigenetic changes in the cells that contribute to malignant transformation and development of cervical cancer. These modifications could be used as biomarkers and new therapeutic molecules that could help in the treatment of cervical cancer.

Conflict of interest

The authors declare no conflict of interest.

Author details

Yair Alfaro-Mora[1], Luis A. Herrera[2], Rodrigo Cáceres-Gutiérrez[2], Marco A. Andonegui-Elguera[2], Guadalupe Dominguez-Gómez[2] and José Díaz-Chávez[2*]

1 Department of Genetics and Molecular Biology, Center for Research and Advanced Studies (CINVESTAV-IPN), Mexico City, México

2 Biomedical Research Unit in Cancer, Biomedical Research Institute, UNAM/ National Cancer Institute (INCan), Mexico City, México

*Address all correspondence to: josediaz030178@hotmail.com

References

[1] Bray F, Ferlay J, Soerjomataram I, Siegel RL, Torre LA, Jemal A. Global cancer statistics 2018: GLOBOCAN estimates of incidence and mortality worldwide for 36 cancers in 185 countries. CA: A Cancer Journal for Clinicians. 2018;**68**(6):394-424

[2] WHO. Cervical Cancer. Geneva: World Health Organization; 2018. Available from: http://www.who.int/cancer/prevention/diagnosis-screening/cervical-cancer/en/

[3] Bruni L, Diaz M, Castellsague X, Ferrer E, Bosch FX, de Sanjose S. Cervical human papillomavirus prevalence in 5 continents: Meta-analysis of 1 million women with normal cytological findings. The Journal of Infectious Diseases. 2010;**202**(12): 1789-1799

[4] Nobbenhuis MA, Helmerhorst TJ, van den Brule AJ, Rozendaal L, Voorhorst FJ, Bezemer PD, et al. Cytological regression and clearance of high-risk human papillomavirus in women with an abnormal cervical smear. Lancet. 2001;**358**(9295): 1782-1783

[5] Schiffman M, Doorbar J, Wentzensen N, de Sanjose S, Fakhry C, Monk BJ, et al. Carcinogenic human papillomavirus infection. Nature Reviews. Disease Primers. 2016;**2**:16086

[6] Pirtea L, Grigoras D, Matusz P, Pirtea M, Moleriu L, Tudor A, et al. Age and HPV type as risk factors for HPV persistence after loop excision in patients with high grade cervical lesions: An observational study. BMC Surgery. 2016;**16**(1):70

[7] Castle PE, Schiffman M, Herrero R, Hildesheim A, Rodriguez AC, Bratti MC, et al. A prospective study of age trends in cervical human papillomavirus acquisition and persistence in Guanacaste, Costa Rica. The Journal of infectious diseases. 2005; **191**(11):1808-1816

[8] International Collaboration of Epidemiological Studies of Cervical Cancer, Appleby P, Beral V, Berrington de Gonzalez A, Colin D, Franceschi S, et al. Carcinoma of the cervix and tobacco smoking: Collaborative reanalysis of individual data on 13,541 women with carcinoma of the cervix and 23,017 women without carcinoma of the cervix from 23 epidemiological studies. International Journal of Cancer. 2006;**118**(6):1481-1495

[9] Marks M, Gravitt PE, Gupta SB, Liaw KL, Tadesse A, Kim E, et al. Combined oral contraceptive use increases HPV persistence but not new HPV detection in a cohort of women from Thailand. The Journal of Infectious Diseases. 2011;**204**(10): 1505-1513

[10] Oh HY, Kim MK, Seo S, Lee DO, Chung YK, Lim MC, et al. Alcohol consumption and persistent infection of high-risk human papillomavirus. Epidemiology and Infection. 2015; **143**(7):1442-1450

[11] Hanahan D, Weinberg RA. Hallmarks of cancer: The next generation. Cell. 2011;**144**(5):646-674

[12] Smith JS, Lindsay L, Hoots B, Keys J, Franceschi S, Winer R, et al. Human papillomavirus type distribution in invasive cervical cancer and high-grade cervical lesions: A meta-analysis update. International Journal of Cancer. 2007; **121**(3):621-632

[13] Doorbar J, Quint W, Banks L, Bravo IG, Stoler M, Broker TR, et al. The biology and life-cycle of human papillomaviruses. Vaccine. 2012;**30** (Suppl 5):F55-F70

[14] Wise-Draper TM, Wells SI. Papillomavirus E6 and E7 proteins and their cellular targets. Frontiers in Bioscience: A Journal and Virtual Library. 2008;**13**:1003-1017

[15] Li C, Fan Y, Li G, Xu X, Duan J, Li R, et al. DNA methylation reprogramming of functional elements during mammalian embryonic development. Cell Discovery. 2018;**4**:41

[16] Gopalakrishnan S, Sullivan BA, Trazzi S, Della Valle G, Robertson KD. DNMT3B interacts with constitutive centromere protein CENP-C to modulate DNA methylation and the histone code at centromeric regions. Human Molecular Genetics. 2009; **18**(17):3178-3193

[17] Sharp AJ, Stathaki E, Migliavacca E, Brahmachary M, Montgomery SB, Dupre Y, et al. DNA methylation profiles of human active and inactive X chromosomes. Genome Research. 2011; **21**(10):1592-1600

[18] Sado T, Okano M, Li E, Sasaki H. De novo DNA methylation is dispensable for the initiation and propagation of X chromosome inactivation. Development. 2004;**131**(5):975-982

[19] Biniszkiewicz D, Gribnau J, Ramsahoye B, Gaudet F, Eggan K, Humpherys D, et al. Dnmt1 overexpression causes genomic hypermethylation, loss of imprinting, and embryonic lethality. Molecular and Cellular Biology. 2002;**22**(7):2124-2135

[20] Xie M, Hong C, Zhang B, Lowdon RF, Xing X, Li D, et al. DNA hypomethylation within specific transposable element families associates with tissue-specific enhancer landscape. Nature Genetics. 2013;**45**(7):836-841

[21] Goll MG, Bestor TH. Eukaryotic cytosine methyltransferases. Annual Review of Biochemistry. 2005;**74**:481-514

[22] Lyko F. The DNA methyltransferase family: A versatile toolkit for epigenetic regulation. Nature Reviews. Genetics. 2018;**19**(2):81-92

[23] Li E, Zhang Y. DNA methylation in mammals. Cold Spring Harbor Perspectives in Biology. 2014;**6**(5): a019133

[24] Jeziorska DM, Murray RJS, De Gobbi M, Gaentzsch R, Garrick D, Ayyub H, et al. DNA methylation of intragenic CpG islands depends on their transcriptional activity during differentiation and disease. Proceedings of the National Academy of Sciences of the United States of America. 2017; **114**(36):E7526-E7E35

[25] Takai D, Jones PA. Comprehensive analysis of CpG islands in human chromosomes 21 and 22. Proceedings of the National Academy of Sciences of the United States of America. 2002;**99**(6): 3740-3745

[26] Gardiner-Garden M, Frommer M. CpG islands in vertebrate genomes. Journal of Molecular Biology. 1987; **196**(2):261-282

[27] Bird A, Taggart M, Frommer M, Miller OJ, Macleod D. A fraction of the mouse genome that is derived from islands of nonmethylated, CpG-rich DNA. Cell. 1985;**40**(1):91-99

[28] Laurent L, Wong E, Li G, Huynh T, Tsirigos A, Ong CT, et al. Dynamic changes in the human methylome during differentiation. Genome Research. 2010;**20**(3):320-331

[29] Wu J, Issa JP, Herman J, Bassett DE Jr, Nelkin BD, Baylin SB. Expression of an exogenous eukaryotic DNA methyltransferase gene induces transformation of NIH 3T3 cells. Proceedings of the National Academy of Sciences of the United States of America. 1993;**90**(19):8891-8895

[30] Sartor MA, Dolinoy DC, Jones TR, Colacino JA, Prince ME, Carey TE, et al. Genome-wide methylation and expression differences in HPV(+) and HPV(−) squamous cell carcinoma cell lines are consistent with divergent mechanisms of carcinogenesis. Epigenetics. 2011;**6**(6):777-787

[31] Sawada M, Kanai Y, Arai E, Ushijima S, Ojima H, Hirohashi S. Increased expression of DNA methyltransferase 1 (DNMT1) protein in uterine cervix squamous cell carcinoma and its precursor lesion. Cancer Letters. 2007;**251**(2):211-219

[32] Leonhardt H, Page AW, Weier HU, Bestor TH. A targeting sequence directs DNA methyltransferase to sites of DNA replication in mammalian nuclei. Cell. 1992;**71**(5):865-873

[33] Okano M, Bell DW, Haber DA, Li E. DNA methyltransferases Dnmt3a and Dnmt3b are essential for de novo methylation and mammalian development. Cell. 1999;**99**(3):247-257

[34] Lin RK, Wu CY, Chang JW, Juan LJ, Hsu HS, Chen CY, et al. Dysregulation of p53/Sp1 control leads to DNA methyltransferase-1 overexpression in lung cancer. Cancer Research. 2010; **70**(14):5807-5817

[35] Au Yeung CL, Tsang WP, Tsang TY, Co NN, Yau PL, Kwok TT. HPV-16 E6 upregulation of DNMT1 through repression of tumor suppressor p53. Oncology Reports. 2010;**24**(6): 1599-1604

[36] D'Costa ZJ, Jolly C, Androphy EJ, Mercer A, Matthews CM, Hibma MH. Transcriptional repression of E-cadherin by human papillomavirus type 16 E6. PLoS One. 2012;**7**(11):e48954

[37] Thomas M, Pim D, Banks L. Human papillomavirus E6 protein interactions. In: McCance DJ, editor. Perspectives in Medical Virology. Vol. 8. Netherlands: Elsevier; 2002. pp. 71-99

[38] Burgers WA, Blanchon L, Pradhan S, de Launoit Y, Kouzarides T, Fuks F. Viral oncoproteins target the DNA methyltransferases. Oncogene. 2007;**26**(11):1650-1655

[39] Laurson J, Khan S, Chung R, Cross K, Raj K. Epigenetic repression of E-cadherin by human papillomavirus 16 E7 protein. Carcinogenesis. 2010;**31**(5): 918-926

[40] McCabe MT, Davis JN, Day ML. Regulation of DNA methyltransferase 1 by the pRb/E2F1 pathway. Cancer Research. 2005;**65**(9):3624-3632

[41] Cicchini L, Blumhagen RZ, Westrich JA, Myers ME, Warren CJ, Siska C, et al. High-risk human papillomavirus E7 alters host DNA methylome and represses HLA-E expression in human keratinocytes. Scientific Reports. 2017;**7**(1):3633

[42] Antinore MJ, Birrer MJ, Patel D, Nader L, McCance DJ. The human papillomavirus type 16 E7 gene product interacts with and trans-activates the AP1 family of transcription factors. The EMBO journal. 1996;**15**(8):1950-1960

[43] Luscher-Firzlaff JM, Westendorf JM, Zwicker J, Burkhardt H, Henriksson M, Muller R, et al. Interaction of the fork head domain transcription factor MPP2 with the human papilloma virus 16 E7 protein: Enhancement of transformation and transactivation. Oncogene. 1999; **18**(41):5620-5630

[44] Hwang SG, Lee D, Kim J, Seo T, Choe J. Human papillomavirus type 16 E7 binds to E2F1 and activates E2F1-driven transcription in a retinoblastoma protein-independent manner. The Journal of Biological Chemistry. 2002; **277**(4):2923-2930

[45] Iliopoulos D, Oikonomou P, Messinis I, Tsezou A. Correlation of promoter hypermethylation in hTERT, DAPK and MGMT genes with cervical oncogenesis progression. Oncology Reports. 2009;**22**(1):199-204

[46] Jeong DH, Youm MY, Kim YN, Lee KB, Sung MS, Yoon HK, et al. Promoter methylation of p16, DAPK, CDH1, and TIMP-3 genes in cervical cancer: Correlation with clinicopathologic characteristics. International Journal of Gynecological Cancer: Official Journal of the International Gynecological Cancer Society. 2006;**16**(3):1234-1240

[47] Ki KD, Lee SK, Tong SY, Lee JM, Song DH, Chi SG. Role of 5'-CpG island hypermethylation of the FHIT gene in cervical carcinoma. Journal of Gynecologic Oncology. 2008;**19**(2): 117-122

[48] Lin Z, Gao M, Zhang X, Kim YS, Lee ES, Kim HK, et al. The hypermethylation and protein expression of p16 INK4A and DNA repair gene O6-methylguanine-DNA methyltransferase in various uterine cervical lesions. Journal of Cancer Research and Clinical Oncology. 2005; **131**(6):364-370

[49] Banzai C, Nishino K, Quan J, Yoshihara K, Sekine M, Yahata T, et al. Promoter methylation of DAPK1, FHIT, MGMT, and CDKN2A genes in cervical carcinoma. International Journal of Clinical Oncology. 2014;**19**(1):127-132

[50] Overmeer RM, Louwers JA, Meijer CJ, van Kemenade FJ, Hesselink AT, Daalmeijer NF, et al. Combined CADM1 and MAL promoter methylation analysis to detect (pre-) malignant cervical lesions in high-risk HPV-positive women. International Journal of Cancer. 2011;**129**(9):2218-2225

[51] Milutin Gasperov N, Sabol I, Planinic P, Grubisic G, Fistonic I, Corusic A, et al. Methylated host cell gene promoters and human papillomavirus type 16 and 18 predicting cervical lesions and cancer. PLoS One. 2015;**10**(6):e0129452

[52] Guerrero-Setas D, Perez-Janices N, Blanco-Fernandez L, Ojer A, Cambra K, Berdasco M, et al. RASSF2 hypermethylation is present and related to shorter survival in squamous cervical cancer. Modern Pathology: An Official Journal of the United States and Canadian Academy of Pathology, Inc. 2013;**26**(8):1111-1122

[53] van der Meide WF, Snellenberg S, Meijer CJ, Baalbergen A, Helmerhorst TJ, van der Sluis WB, et al. Promoter methylation analysis of WNT/beta-catenin signaling pathway regulators to detect adenocarcinoma or its precursor lesion of the cervix. Gynecologic Oncology. 2011;**123**(1): 116-122

[54] Steenbergen RD, Ongenaert M, Snellenberg S, Trooskens G, van der Meide WF, Pandey D, et al. Methylation-specific digital karyotyping of HPV16E6E7-expressing human keratinocytes identifies novel methylation events in cervical carcinogenesis. The Journal of Pathology. 2013;**231**(1):53-62

[55] Song Y, Zhang C. Hydralazine inhibits human cervical cancer cell growth in vitro in association with APC demethylation and re-expression. Cancer Chemotherapy and Pharmacology. 2009;**63**(4):605-613

[56] Sova P, Feng Q, Geiss G, Wood T, Strauss R, Rudolf V, et al. Discovery of novel methylation biomarkers in cervical carcinoma by global demethylation and microarray analysis. Cancer Epidemiology, Biomarkers and Prevention: A Publication of the American Association for Cancer Research, cosponsored by the American

Society of Preventive Oncology. 2006; **15**(1):114-123

[57] Li L, Xu C, Long J, Shen D, Zhou W, Zhou Q, et al. E6 and E7 gene silencing results in decreased methylation of tumor suppressor genes and induces phenotype transformation of human cervical carcinoma cell lines. Oncotarget. 2015;**6**(27):23930-23943

[58] Chalertpet K, Pakdeechaidan W, Patel V, Mutirangura A, Yanatatsaneejit P. Human papillomavirus type 16 E7 oncoprotein mediates CCNA1 promoter methylation. Cancer Science. 2015;**106**(10):1333-1340

[59] Zhang Y, Chen FQ, Sun YH, Zhou SY, Li TY, Chen R. Effects of DNMT1 silencing on malignant phenotype and methylated gene expression in cervical cancer cells. Journal of Experimental and Clinical Cancer Research. 2011;**30**:98

[60] Feng Q, Balasubramanian A, Hawes SE, Toure P, Sow PS, Dem A, et al. Detection of hypermethylated genes in women with and without cervical neoplasia. Journal of the National Cancer Institute. 2005;**97**(4): 273-282

[61] Holubekova V, Mendelova A, Grendar M, Mersakova S, Kapustova I, Jasek K, et al. Methylation pattern of CDH1 promoter and its association with CDH1 gene expression in cytological cervical specimens. Oncology Letters. 2016;**12**(4):2613-2621

[62] Jha S, Vande Pol S, Banerjee NS, Dutta AB, Chow LT, Dutta A. Destabilization of TIP60 by human papillomavirus E6 results in attenuation of TIP60-dependent transcriptional regulation and apoptotic pathway. Molecular Cell. 2010;**38**(5):700-711

[63] Yang HJ, Liu VW, Wang Y, Tsang PC, Ngan HY. Differential DNA methylation profiles in gynecological cancers and correlation with clinico-pathological data. BMC Cancer. 2006;**6**: 212

[64] Liu L, Zhang J, Bates S, Li JJ, Peehl DM, Rhim JS, et al. A methylation profile of in vitro immortalized human cell lines. International Journal of Oncology. 2005;**26**(1):275-285

[65] Cicchini L, Westrich JA, Xu T, Vermeer DW, Berger JN, Clambey ET, et al. Suppression of antitumor immune responses by human papillomavirus through epigenetic downregulation of CXCL14. MBio. 2016;**7**(3)

[66] Cohen Y, Singer G, Lavie O, Dong SM, Beller U, Sidransky D. The RASSF1A tumor suppressor gene is commonly inactivated in adenocarcinoma of the uterine cervix. Clinical Cancer Research: An Official Journal of the American Association for Cancer Research. 2003;**9**(8):2981-2984

[67] Widschwendter A, Ivarsson L, Blassnig A, Muller HM, Fiegl H, Wiedemair A, et al. CDH1 and CDH13 methylation in serum is an independent prognostic marker in cervical cancer patients. International Journal of Cancer. 2004;**109**(2):163-166

[68] Huang Y, Song H, Hu H, Cui L, You C, Huang L. Trichosanthin inhibits DNA methyltransferase and restores methylation-silenced gene expression in human cervical cancer cells. Molecular Medicine Reports. 2012;**6**(4):872-878

[69] Starnes T, Rasila KK, Robertson MJ, Brahmi Z, Dahl R, Christopherson K, et al. The chemokine CXCL14 (BRAK) stimulates activated NK cell migration: Implications for the downregulation of CXCL14 in malignancy. Experimental Hematology. 2006;**34**(8):1101-1105

[70] Shellenberger TD, Wang M, Gujrati M, Jayakumar A, Strieter RM, Burdick MD, et al. BRAK/CXCL14 is a

potent inhibitor of angiogenesis and a chemotactic factor for immature dendritic cells. Cancer Research. 2004; **64**(22):8262-8270

[71] Matthews K, Leong CM, Baxter L, Inglis E, Yun K, Backstrom BT, et al. Depletion of Langerhans cells in human papillomavirus type 16-infected skin is associated with E6-mediated down regulation of E-cadherin. Journal of Virology. 2003;**77**(15):8378-8385

[72] Cao Q, Yu J, Dhanasekaran SM, Kim JH, Mani RS, Tomlins SA, et al. Repression of E-cadherin by the polycomb group protein EZH2 in cancer. Oncogene. 2008;**27**(58):7274-7284

[73] Wang C, Liu X, Chen Z, Huang H, Jin Y, Kolokythas A, et al. Polycomb group protein EZH2-mediated E-cadherin repression promotes metastasis of oral tongue squamous cell carcinoma. Molecular Carcinogenesis. 2013;**52**(3): 229-236

[74] Holland D, Hoppe-Seyler K, Schuller B, Lohrey C, Maroldt J, Durst M, et al. Activation of the enhancer of zeste homologue 2 gene by the human papillomavirus E7 oncoprotein. Cancer Research. 2008;**68**(23):9964-9972

[75] van der Vlag J, Otte AP. Transcriptional repression mediated by the human polycomb-group protein EED involves histone deacetylation. Nature Genetics. 1999;**23**(4):474-478

[76] Kleer CG, Cao Q, Varambally S, Shen R, Ota I, Tomlins SA, et al. EZH2 is a marker of aggressive breast cancer and promotes neoplastic transformation of breast epithelial cells. Proceedings of the National Academy of Sciences of the United States of America. 2003; **100**(20):11606-11611

[77] Bodily JM, Mehta KP, Laimins LA. Human papillomavirus E7 enhances hypoxia-inducible factor 1-mediated transcription by inhibiting binding of histone deacetylases. Cancer Research. 2011;**71**(3):1187-1195

[78] Sun NX, Ye C, Zhao Q, Zhang Q, Xu C, Wang SB, et al. Long noncoding RNA-EBIC promotes tumor cell invasion by binding to EZH2 and repressing E-cadherin in cervical cancer. PLoS One. 2014;**9**(7):e100340

[79] He H, Liu X, Liu Y, Zhang M, Lai Y, Hao Y, et al. Human papillomavirus E6/ E7 and long noncoding RNA TMPOP2 mutually upregulated gene expression in cervical cancer cells. Journal of Virology. 2019;**93**(8)

[80] Samuelsson J, Alonso S, Ruiz-Larroya T, Cheung TH, Wong YF, Perucho M. Frequent somatic demethylation of RAPGEF1/C3G intronic sequences in gastrointestinal and gynecological cancer. International Journal of Oncology. 2011;**38**(6): 1575-1577

[81] Lee TS, Kim JW, Kang GH, Park NH, Song YS, Kang SB, et al. DNA hypomethylation of CAGE promotors in squamous cell carcinoma of uterine cervix. Annals of the New York Academy of Sciences. 2006;**1091**: 218-224

[82] Yin FF, Wang N, Bi XN, Yu X, Xu XH, Wang YL, et al. Serine/ threonine kinases 31(STK31) may be a novel cellular target gene for the HPV16 oncogene E7 with potential as a DNA hypomethylation biomarker in cervical cancer. Virology Journal. 2016;**13**:60

[83] Thangavelu PU, Krenacs T, Dray E, Duijf PH. In epithelial cancers, aberrant COL17A1 promoter methylation predicts its misexpression and increased invasion. Clinical Epigenetics. 2016;**8**:120

[84] Zhou H, Wang Y, Lv Q, Zhang J, Wang Q, Gao F, et al. Overexpression of

ribosomal RNA in the development of human cervical cancer is associated with rDNA promoter hypomethylation. PLoS One. 2016;**11**(10):e0163340

[85] Stunkel W, Bernard HU. The chromatin structure of the long control region of human papillomavirus type 16 represses viral oncoprotein expression. Journal of Virology. 1999;**73**(3): 1918-1930

[86] Favre M, Breitburd F, Croissant O, Orth G. Chromatin-like structures obtained after alkaline disruption of bovine and human papillomaviruses. Journal of Virology. 1977;**21**(3): 1205-1209

[87] Thierry F, Yaniv M. The BPV1-E2 trans-acting protein can be either an activator or a repressor of the HPV18 regulatory region. The EMBO Journal. 1987;**6**(11):3391-3397

[88] Steger G, Corbach S. Dose-dependent regulation of the early promoter of human papillomavirus type 18 by the viral E2 protein. Journal of Virology. 1997;**71**(1):50-58

[89] Romanczuk H, Thierry F, Howley PM. Mutational analysis of cis elements involved in E2 modulation of human papillomavirus type 16 P97 and type 18 P105 promoters. Journal of Virology. 1990;**64**(6):2849-2859

[90] Schwarz E, Freese UK, Gissmann L, Mayer W, Roggenbuck B, Stremlau A, et al. Structure and transcription of human papillomavirus sequences in cervical carcinoma cells. Nature. 1985; **314**(6006):111-114

[91] Demeret C, Desaintes C, Yaniv M, Thierry F. Different mechanisms contribute to the E2-mediated transcriptional repression of human papillomavirus type 18 viral oncogenes. Journal of Virology. 1997;**71**(12): 9343-9349

[92] Wu SY, Lee AY, Hou SY, Kemper JK, Erdjument-Bromage H, Tempst P, et al. Brd4 links chromatin targeting to HPV transcriptional silencing. Genes and Development. 2006;**20**(17):2383-2396

[93] Yan J, Li Q, Lievens S, Tavernier J, You J. Abrogation of the Brd4-positive transcription elongation factor B complex by papillomavirus E2 protein contributes to viral oncogene repression. Journal of Virology. 2010; **84**(1):76-87

[94] Romanczuk H, Howley PM. Disruption of either the E1 or the E2 regulatory gene of human papillomavirus type 16 increases viral immortalization capacity. Proceedings of the National Academy of Sciences of the United States of America. 1992; **89**(7):3159-3163

[95] Chaiwongkot A, Vinokurova S, Pientong C, Ekalaksananan T, Kongyingyoes B, Kleebkaow P, et al. Differential methylation of E2 binding sites in episomal and integrated HPV 16 genomes in preinvasive and invasive cervical lesions. International Journal of Cancer. 2013;**132**(9):2087-2094

[96] McBride AA, Warburton A. The role of integration in oncogenic progression of HPV-associated cancers. PLoS Pathogens. 2017;**13**(4): e1006211

[97] Vinokurova S, von Knebel Doeberitz M. Differential methylation of the HPV 16 upstream regulatory region during epithelial differentiation and neoplastic transformation. PLoS One. 2011;**6**(9):e24451

[98] Bhattacharjee B, Sengupta S. CpG methylation of HPV 16 LCR at E2 binding site proximal to P97 is associated with cervical cancer in presence of intact E2. Virology. 2006; **354**(2):280-285

[99] Thain A, Jenkins O, Clarke AR, Gaston K. CpG methylation directly inhibits binding of the human papillomavirus type 16 E2 protein to specific DNA sequences. Journal of Virology. 1996;**70**(10):7233-7235

[100] Kim K, Garner-Hamrick PA, Fisher C, Lee D, Lambert PF. Methylation patterns of papillomavirus DNA, its influence on E2 function, and implications in viral infection. Journal of Virology. 2003;**77**(23):12450-12459

[101] McAnena P, Brown JA, Kerin MJ. Circulating nucleosomes and nucleosome modifications as biomarkers in cancer. Cancers. 2017;**9**(1)

[102] Chen Y, Sprung R, Tang Y, Ball H, Sangras B, Kim SC, et al. Lysine propionylation and butyrylation are novel post-translational modifications in histones. Molecular and Cellular Proteomics—MCP. 2007;**6**(5):812-819

[103] Hasan UA, Zannetti C, Parroche P, Goutagny N, Malfroy M, Roblot G, et al. The human papillomavirus type 16 E7 oncoprotein induces a transcriptional repressor complex on the toll-like receptor 9 promoter. The Journal of Experimental Medicine. 2013;**210**(7):1369-1387

[104] Karim R, Meyers C, Backendorf C, Ludigs K, Offringa R, van Ommen GJ, et al. Human papillomavirus deregulates the response of a cellular network comprising of chemotactic and proinflammatory genes. PLoS One. 2011;**6**(3):e17848

[105] Andersen JM, Al-Khairy D, Ingalls RR. Innate immunity at the mucosal surface: Role of toll-like receptor 3 and toll-like receptor 9 in cervical epithelial cell responses to microbial pathogens. Biology of Reproduction. 2006;**74**(5):824-831

[106] Cannella F, Pierangeli A, Scagnolari C, Cacciotti G, Tranquilli G, Stentella P, et al. TLR9 is expressed in human papillomavirus-positive cervical cells and is overexpressed in persistent infections. Immunobiology. 2015; **220**(3):363-368

[107] Tanaka N, Kawakami T, Taniguchi T. Recognition DNA sequences of interferon regulatory factor 1 (IRF-1) and IRF-2, regulators of cell growth and the interferon system. Molecular and Cellular Biology. 1993;**13**(8):4531-4538

[108] Yanai H, Negishi H, Taniguchi T. The IRF family of transcription factors: Inception, impact and implications in oncogenesis. Oncoimmunology. 2012; **1**(8):1376-1386

[109] Brehm A, Nielsen SJ, Miska EA, McCance DJ, Reid JL, Bannister AJ, et al. The E7 oncoprotein associates with Mi2 and histone deacetylase activity to promote cell growth. The EMBO Journal. 1999;**18**(9):2449-2458

[110] Park JS, Kim EJ, Kwon HJ, Hwang ES, Namkoong SE, Um SJ. Inactivation of interferon regulatory factor-1 tumor suppressor protein by HPV E7 oncoprotein. Implication for the E7-mediated immune evasion mechanism in cervical carcinogenesis. The Journal of Biological Chemistry. 2000;**275**(10):6764-6769

[111] Sheppard KA, Rose DW, Haque ZK, Kurokawa R, McInerney E, Westin S, et al. Transcriptional activation by NF-kappaB requires multiple coactivators. Molecular and Cellular Biology. 1999;**19**(9):6367-6378

[112] Zhong H, Voll RE, Ghosh S. Phosphorylation of NF-kappa B p65 by PKA stimulates transcriptional activity by promoting a novel bivalent interaction with the coactivator CBP/ p300. Molecular Cell. 1998;**1**(5):661-671

[113] Giebler HA, Lemasson I, Nyborg JK. p53 recruitment of CREB binding protein mediated through phosphorylated CREB: A novel pathway

of tumor suppressor regulation. Molecular and Cellular Biology. 2000; **20**(13):4849-4858

[114] An W, Kim J, Roeder RG. Ordered cooperative functions of PRMT1, p300, and CARM1 in transcriptional activation by p53. Cell. 2004;**117**(6):735-748

[115] Jin Q, Yu LR, Wang L, Zhang Z, Kasper LH, Lee JE, et al. Distinct roles of GCN5/PCAF-mediated H3K9ac and CBP/p300-mediated H3K18/27ac in nuclear receptor transactivation. The EMBO Journal. 2011;**30**(2):249-262

[116] Hennig AK, Peng GH, Chen S. Transcription coactivators p300 and CBP are necessary for photoreceptor-specific chromatin organization and gene expression. PLoS One. 2013;**8**(7):e69721

[117] Raisner R, Kharbanda S, Jin L, Jeng E, Chan E, Merchant M, et al. Enhancer activity requires CBP/P300 bromodomain-dependent histone H3K27 acetylation. Cell Reports. 2018; **24**(7):1722-1729

[118] Ramos YF, Hestand MS, Verlaan M, Krabbendam E, Ariyurek Y, van Galen M, et al. Genome-wide assessment of differential roles for p300 and CBP in transcription regulation. Nucleic Acids Research. 2010;**38**(16):5396-5408

[119] Zhang Q, Vo N, Goodman RH. Histone binding protein RbAp48 interacts with a complex of CREB binding protein and phosphorylated CREB. Molecular and Cellular Biology. 2000;**20**(14):4970-4978

[120] Ito T, Ikehara T, Nakagawa T, Kraus WL, Muramatsu M. p300-mediated acetylation facilitates the transfer of histone H2A-H2B dimers from nucleosomes to a histone chaperone. Genes and Development. 2000;**14**(15):1899-1907

[121] Ito A, Lai CH, Zhao X, Saito S, Hamilton MH, Appella E, et al. p300/CBP-mediated p53 acetylation is commonly induced by p53-activating agents and inhibited by MDM2. The EMBO Journal. 2001;**20**(6):1331-1340

[122] Hsu CH, Peng KL, Jhang HC, Lin CH, Wu SY, Chiang CM, et al. The HPV E6 oncoprotein targets histone methyltransferases for modulating specific gene transcription. Oncogene. 2012;**31**(18):2335-2349

[123] Avantaggiati ML, Ogryzko V, Gardner K, Giordano A, Levine AS, Kelly K. Recruitment of p300/CBP in p53-dependent signal pathways. Cell. 1997;**89**(7):1175-1184

[124] Gu W, Shi XL, Roeder RG. Synergistic activation of transcription by CBP and p53. Nature. 1997; **387**(6635):819-823

[125] Van Orden K, Giebler HA, Lemasson I, Gonzales M, Nyborg JK. Binding of p53 to the KIX domain of CREB binding protein. A potential link to human T-cell leukemia virus, type I-associated leukemogenesis. The Journal of Biological Chemistry. 1999;**274**(37): 26321-26328

[126] Grossman SR, Perez M, Kung AL, Joseph M, Mansur C, Xiao ZX, et al. p300/MDM2 complexes participate in MDM2-mediated p53 degradation. Molecular Cell. 1998;**2**(4):405-415

[127] Teufel DP, Freund SM, Bycroft M, Fersht AR. Four domains of p300 each bind tightly to a sequence spanning both transactivation subdomains of p53. Proceedings of the National Academy of Sciences of the United States of America. 2007;**104**(17):7009-7014

[128] Gu W, Roeder RG. Activation of p53 sequence-specific DNA binding by acetylation of the p53 C-terminal domain. Cell. 1997;**90**(4):595-606

[129] Thomas MC, Chiang CM. E6 oncoprotein represses p53-dependent

gene activation via inhibition of protein acetylation independently of inducing p53 degradation. Molecular Cell. 2005; **17**(2):251-264

[130] Lee CW, Ferreon JC, Ferreon AC, Arai M, Wright PE. Graded enhancement of p53 binding to CREB-binding protein (CBP) by multisite phosphorylation. Proceedings of the National Academy of Sciences of the United States of America. 2010;**107**(45): 19290-19295

[131] Zimmermann H, Degenkolbe R, Bernard HU, O'Connor MJ. The human papillomavirus type 16 E6 oncoprotein can down-regulate p53 activity by targeting the transcriptional coactivator CBP/p300. Journal of Virology. 1999; **73**(8):6209-6219

[132] Esteve PO, Chin HG, Benner J, Feehery GR, Samaranayake M, Horwitz GA, et al. Regulation of DNMT1 stability through SET7-mediated lysine methylation in mammalian cells. Proceedings of the National Academy of Sciences of the United States of America. 2009;**106**(13):5076-5081

[133] Patel D, Huang SM, Baglia LA, McCance DJ. The E6 protein of human papillomavirus type 16 binds to and inhibits co-activation by CBP and p300. The EMBO Journal. 1999;**18**(18): 5061-5072

[134] Huang SM, McCance DJ. Down regulation of the interleukin-8 promoter by human papillomavirus type 16 E6 and E7 through effects on CREB binding protein/p300 and P/CAF. Journal of Virology. 2002;**76**(17): 8710-8721

[135] Avvakumov N, Torchia J, Mymryk JS. Interaction of the HPV E7 proteins with the pCAF acetyltransferase. Oncogene. 2003; **22**(25):3833-3841

[136] Bernat A, Massimi P, Banks L. Complementation of a p300/CBP defective-binding mutant of adenovirus E1a by human papillomavirus E6 proteins. The Journal of General Virology. 2002;**83**(Pt 4):829-833

[137] Jansma AL, Martinez-Yamout MA, Liao R, Sun P, Dyson HJ, Wright PE. The high-risk HPV16 E7 oncoprotein mediates interaction between the transcriptional coactivator CBP and the retinoblastoma protein pRb. Journal of Molecular Biology. 2014;**426**(24): 4030-4048

[138] Hangauer MJ, Vaughn IW, McManus MT. Pervasive transcription of the human genome produces thousands of previously unidentified long intergenic noncoding RNAs. PLoS Genetics. 2013;**9**(6):e1003569

[139] Djebali S, Davis CA, Merkel A, Dobin A, Lassmann T, Mortazavi A, et al. Landscape of transcription in human cells. Nature. 2012;**489**(7414): 101-108

[140] Guennewig B, Cooper AA. The central role of noncoding RNA in the brain. International Review of Neurobiology. 2014;**116**:153-194

[141] Pereira PM, Marques JP, Soares AR, Carreto L, Santos MA. MicroRNA expression variability in human cervical tissues. PLoS One. 2010; **5**(7):e11780

[142] Chen Y, Wang CX, Sun XX, Wang C, Liu TF, Wang DJ. Long non-coding RNA CCHE1 overexpression predicts a poor prognosis for cervical cancer. European Review for Medical and Pharmacological Sciences. 2017; **21**(3):479-483

[143] Yang M, Zhai X, Xia B, Wang Y, Lou G. Long noncoding RNA CCHE1 promotes cervical cancer cell proliferation via upregulating PCNA.

Tumour Biology: Journal of the International Society for Oncodevelopmental Biology and Medicine. 2015;**36**(10):7615-7622

[144] Barr JA, Hayes KE, Brownmiller T, Harold AD, Jagannathan R, Lockman PR, et al. Long non-coding RNA FAM83H-AS1 is regulated by human papillomavirus 16 E6 independently of p53 in cervical cancer cells. Scientific Reports. 2019;**9**(1):3662

[145] Lui WO, Pourmand N, Patterson BK, Fire A. Patterns of known and novel small RNAs in human cervical cancer. Cancer Research. 2007;**67**(13):6031-6043

[146] Cao S, Liu W, Li F, Zhao W, Qin C. Decreased expression of lncRNA GAS5 predicts a poor prognosis in cervical cancer. International Journal of Clinical and Experimental Pathology. 2014;**7**(10):6776-6783

[147] Hu X, Schwarz JK, Lewis JS Jr, Huettner PC, Rader JS, Deasy JO, et al. A microRNA expression signature for cervical cancer prognosis. Cancer Research. 2010;**70**(4):1441-1448

[148] Kim SJ, Park SE, Lee C, Lee SY, Jo JH, Kim JM, et al. Alterations in promoter usage and expression levels of insulin-like growth factor-II and H19 genes in cervical carcinoma exhibiting biallelic expression of IGF-II. Biochimica et Biophysica Acta. 2002;**1586**(3):307-315

[149] Sharma S, Mandal P, Sadhukhan T, Roy Chowdhury R, Ranjan Mondal N, Chakravarty B, et al. Bridging links between long noncoding RNA HOTAIR and HPV oncoprotein E7 in cervical cancer pathogenesis. Scientific Reports. 2015;**5**:11724

[150] Sehnal B, Zikan M, Nipcova M, Dusek L, Cibula D, Slama J. The association among cervical, anal, and oral HPV infections in high-risk and low-risk women. European Journal of Obstetrics and Gynecology and Reproductive Biology. 2019;**4**:100061

[151] Jiang S, Wang HL, Yang J. Low expression of long non-coding RNA LET inhibits carcinogenesis of cervical cancer. International Journal of Clinical and Experimental Pathology. 2015;**8**(1):806-811

[152] Jiang Y, Li Y, Fang S, Jiang B, Qin C, Xie P, et al. The role of MALAT1 correlates with HPV in cervical cancer. Oncology Letters. 2014;**7**(6):2135-2141

[153] Zhang J, Yao T, Wang Y, Yu J, Liu Y, Lin Z. Long noncoding RNA MEG3 is downregulated in cervical cancer and affects cell proliferation and apoptosis by regulating miR-21. Cancer Biology and Therapy. 2016;**17**(1):104-113

[154] Qin R, Chen Z, Ding Y, Hao J, Hu J, Guo F. Long non-coding RNA MEG3 inhibits the proliferation of cervical carcinoma cells through the induction of cell cycle arrest and apoptosis. Neoplasma. 2013;**60**(5):486-492

[155] Zhou D, Wu F, Cui Y, Wei F, Meng Q, Lv Q. Long non-coding RNA-OIS1 inhibits HPV-positive, but not HPV-negative cervical squamous cell carcinoma by upregulating MTK-1. Oncology Letters. 2019;**17**(3):2923-2930

[156] Iden M, Fye S, Li K, Chowdhury T, Ramchandran R, Rader JS. The lncRNA PVT1 contributes to the cervical cancer phenotype and associates with poor patient prognosis. PLoS One. 2016;**11**(5):e0156274

[157] Liu Q, Guo X, Que S, Yang X, Fan H, Liu M, et al. LncRNA RSU1P2 contributes to tumorigenesis by acting as a ceRNA against let-7a in cervical cancer cells. Oncotarget. 2017;**8**(27):43768-43781

[158] Kang HW, Wang F, Wei Q, Zhao YF, Liu M, Li X, et al. miR-20a promotes migration and invasion by regulating TNKS2 in human cervical cancer cells. FEBS Letters. 2012;**586**(6): 897-904

[159] Cao Y, Liu Y, Lu X, Wang Y, Qiao H, Liu M. Upregulation of long noncoding RNA SPRY4-IT1 correlates with tumor progression and poor prognosis in cervical cancer. FEBS Open Bio. 2016;**6**(9):954-960

[160] Chen X, Liu L, Zhu W. Up-regulation of long non-coding RNA CCAT2 correlates with tumor metastasis and poor prognosis in cervical squamous cell cancer patients. International Journal of Clinical and Experimental Pathology. 2015;**8**(10):13261-13266

[161] Wu L, Jin L, Zhang W, Zhang L. Roles of long non-coding RNA CCAT2 in cervical cancer cell growth and apoptosis. Medical Science Monitor: International Medical Journal of Experimental and Clinical Research. 2016;**22**:875-879

[162] Kawakami T, Zhang C, Taniguchi T, Kim CJ, Okada Y, Sugihara H, et al. Characterization of loss-of-inactive X in Klinefelter syndrome and female-derived cancer cells. Oncogene. 2004;**23**(36):6163-6169

[163] Sharma S, Munger K. Expression of the cervical carcinoma expressed PCNA regulatory (CCEPR) long noncoding RNA is driven by the human papillomavirus E6 protein and modulates cell proliferation independent of PCNA. Virology. 2018;**518**:8-13

[164] Liao LM, Sun XY, Liu AW, Wu JB, Cheng XL, Lin JX, et al. Low expression of long noncoding XLOC_010588 indicates a poor prognosis and promotes proliferation through upregulation of c-Myc in cervical cancer. Gynecologic Oncology. 2014;**133**(3):616-623

[165] Lee JW, Choi CH, Choi JJ, Park YA, Kim SJ, Hwang SY, et al. Altered microRNA expression in cervical carcinomas. Clinical Cancer Research: An Official Journal of the American Association for Cancer Research. 2008; **14**(9):2535-2542

[166] Wang X, Tang S, Le SY, Lu R, Rader JS, Meyers C, et al. Aberrant expression of oncogenic and tumor-suppressive microRNAs in cervical cancer is required for cancer cell growth. PLoS One. 2008;**3**(7):e2557

[167] Li Y, Wang F, Xu J, Ye F, Shen Y, Zhou J, et al. Progressive miRNA expression profiles in cervical carcinogenesis and identification of HPV-related target genes for miR-29. The Journal of pathology. 2011;**224**(4): 484-495

[168] Lajer CB, Garnaes E, Friis-Hansen L, Norrild B, Therkildsen MH, Glud M, et al. The role of miRNAs in human papilloma virus (HPV)-associated cancers: Bridging between HPV-related head and neck cancer and cervical cancer. British Journal of Cancer. 2012; **106**(9):1526-1534

[169] Liu S, Song L, Zeng S, Zhang L. MALAT1-miR-124-RBG2 axis is involved in growth and invasion of HR-HPV-positive cervical cancer cells. Tumour Biology: Journal of the International Society for Oncodevelopmental Biology and Medicine. 2016;**37**(1):633-640

[170] Martinez I, Gardiner AS, Board KF, Monzon FA, Edwards RP, Khan SA. Human papillomavirus type 16 reduces the expression of microRNA-218 in cervical carcinoma cells. Oncogene. 2008;**27**(18):2575-2582

[171] Xu Z, Zhou Y, Shi F, Cao Y, Dinh TLA, Wan J, et al. Investigation of differentially-expressed microRNAs and genes in cervical cancer using an

integrated bioinformatics analysis. Oncology Letters. 2017;**13**(4):2784-2790

[172] Gardiner AS, McBee WC, Edwards RP, Austin M, Lesnock JL, Bhargava R, et al. MicroRNA analysis in human papillomavirus (HPV)-associated cervical neoplasia and cancer. Infectious Agents and Cancer. 2010; **5**(1):A55

[173] Bodaghi S, Jia R, Zheng ZM. Human papillomavirus type 16 E2 and E6 are RNA-binding proteins and inhibit in vitro splicing of pre-mRNAs with suboptimal splice sites. Virology. 2009;**386**(1):32-43

[174] Yeung CL, Tsang TY, Yau PL, Kwok TT. Human papillomavirus type 16 E6 suppresses microRNA-23b expression in human cervical cancer cells through DNA methylation of the host gene C9orf3. Oncotarget. 2017; **8**(7):12158-12173

[175] Jung HM, Phillips BL, Chan EK. miR-375 activates p21 and suppresses telomerase activity by coordinately regulating HPV E6/E7, E6AP, CIP2A, and 14-3-3zeta. Molecular Cancer. 2014; **13**:80

[176] Morel A, Baguet A, Perrard J, Demeret C, Jacquin E, Guenat D, et al. 5azadC treatment upregulates miR-375 level and represses HPV16 E6 expression. Oncotarget. 2017;**8**(28): 46163-46176

[177] Wang F, Li Y, Zhou J, Xu J, Peng C, Ye F, et al. miR-375 is down-regulated in squamous cervical cancer and inhibits cell migration and invasion via targeting transcription factor SP1. The American Journal of Pathology. 2011;**179**(5): 2580-2588

[178] Liu S, Song L, Yao H, Zhang L, Xu D, Gao F, et al. MiR-375 is epigenetically downregulated by HPV-16 E6 mediated DNMT1 upregulation and modulates EMT of cervical cancer cells by suppressing lncRNA MALAT1. PLoS One. 2016;**11**(9):e0163460

[179] Khalil AM, Guttman M, Huarte M, Garber M, Raj A, Rivea Morales D, et al. Many human large intergenic noncoding RNAs associate with chromatin-modifying complexes and affect gene expression. Proceedings of the National Academy of Sciences of the United States of America. 2009;**106**(28): 11667-11672

[180] Lu H, He Y, Lin L, Qi Z, Ma L, Li L, et al. Long non-coding RNA MALAT1 modulates radiosensitivity of HR-HPV+ cervical cancer via sponging miR-145. Tumour Biology: Journal of the International Society for Oncodevelopmental Biology and Medicine. 2016;**37**(2):1683-1691

[181] Rinn JL, Kertesz M, Wang JK, Squazzo SL, Xu X, Brugmann SA, et al. Functional demarcation of active and silent chromatin domains in human HOX loci by noncoding RNAs. Cell. 2007;**129**(7):1311-1323

[182] Gupta RA, Shah N, Wang KC, Kim J, Horlings HM, Wong DJ, et al. Long non-coding RNA HOTAIR reprograms chromatin state to promote cancer metastasis. Nature. 2010; **464**(7291):1071-1076

[183] Zhang M, Song Y, Zhai F. ARFHPV E7 oncogene, lncRNA HOTAIR, miR-331-3p and its target, NRP2, form a negative feedback loop to regulate the apoptosis in the tumorigenesis in HPV positive cervical cancer. Journal of Cellular Biochemistry. 2018;**119**(6):4397-4407

[184] Fujii T, Shimada K, Asano A, Tatsumi Y, Yamaguchi N, Yamazaki M, et al. MicroRNA-331-3p suppresses cervical cancer cell proliferation and E6/ E7 expression by targeting NRP2. International Journal of Molecular Sciences. 2016;**17**(8)

[185] Zambrano P, Segura-Pacheco B, Perez-Cardenas E, Cetina L, Revilla-Vazquez A, Taja-Chayeb L, et al. A phase I study of hydralazine to demethylate and reactivate the expression of tumor suppressor genes. BMC Cancer. 2005;**5**:44

[186] de la Cruz-Hernandez E, Perez-Cardenas E, Contreras-Paredes A, Cantu D, Mohar A, Lizano M, et al. The effects of DNA methylation and histone deacetylase inhibitors on human papillomavirus early gene expression in cervical cancer, an in vitro and clinical study. Virology Journal. 2007;**4**:18

[187] You JS, Kang JK, Lee EK, Lee JC, Lee SH, Jeon YJ, et al. Histone deacetylase inhibitor apicidin downregulates DNA methyltransferase 1 expression and induces repressive histone modifications via recruitment of corepressor complex to promoter region in human cervix cancer cells. Oncogene. 2008;**27**(10):1376-1386

[188] Li Y, Yao J, Han C, Yang J, Chaudhry MT, Wang S, et al. Quercetin, inflammation and immunity. Nutrients. 2016;**8**(3):167

[189] Kedhari Sundaram M, Hussain A, Haque S, Raina R, Afroze N. Quercetin modifies 5'CpG promoter methylation and reactivates various tumor suppressor genes by modulating epigenetic marks in human cervical cancer cells. Journal of Cellular Biochemistry. 2019

[190] Lewis A, Kang R, Levine A, Maghami E. The new face of head and neck cancer: The HPV epidemic. Oncology. 2015;**29**(9):616-626

[191] Kim SM. Human papilloma virus in oral cancer. Journal of the Korean Association of Oral and Maxillofacial Surgeons. 2016;**42**(6):327-336

[192] Hernandez BY, McDuffie K, Zhu X, Wilkens LR, Killeen J, Kessel B, et al. Anal human papillomavirus infection in women and its relationship with cervical infection. Cancer Epidemiology, Biomarkers and Prevention: A Publication of the American Association for Cancer Research, Cosponsored by the American Society of Preventive Oncology. 2005;**14**(11 Pt 1):2550-2556

Chapter 3

Glucagonoma Masquerading as a Mucinous Cancer of the Ovary: Lessons from Cell Biology

Gwo Yaw Ho, Sumitra Ananda, Cassandra J. Vandenberg, Orla McNally, Jeanne Tie, Kylie Gorringe, David Bowtell, Jan Pyman, Matthew J. Wakefield and Clare L. Scott

Abstract

High-grade mucinous ovarian cancer (HGMOC) is often a misnomer as the majority of cases are metastatic disease with a gastro-intestinal origin. The standard platinum-based ovarian cancer (OC) chemotherapy regimens are often ineffective, and there are insufficient data to support the use of colorectal cancer (CRC) chemotherapy regimens due to the rarity of HGMOC. We described a cohort of four consecutive suspected HGMOC cases treated at the Royal Women's Hospital, Melbourne in 2012. Two cases were treated as primary MOC, whereas the other two were considered to be metastatic CRC based on histopathological and clinical evidence. From the RNAseq analysis, we identified two cases of HGMOC whose gene expression profiles were consistent with mucinous epithelial OC, one case that was treated as metastatic CRC with gene expression profile correlated with CRC and one case with neuroendocrine (NET) gene expression features. Interestingly, glucagon was over-expressed in this tumor that was subsequently confirmed by immunohistochemistry. These findings suggest a rare glucagonoma-like NET appendiceal tumor that had metastasized to the surface of ovary and were unresponsive to CRC chemotherapy regimens. In summary, a carefully curated panel of expression markers and selected functional genomics could provide diagnosis and treatment guidance for patients with possible HGMOC.

Keywords: mucinous ovarian cancer, glucagonoma, genomic

1. Introduction

Primary mucinous epithelial ovarian cancer (mEOC) is a rare subset, 2.7–11.9%, of epithelial ovarian cancer. The incidence for high grade mucinous ovarian cancer (HGMOC) is even lower [1]. More than two-thirds of primary HGMOC cases are misdiagnoses, which has huge implications for the outcome of these patients [2]. The overall 5-year survival outcome for localised primary mucinous ovarian cancer is over 95%, whereas the life expectancy of women with metastatic mucinous cancer ranges from months to years depending on the organ site of the primary tumour. Primary mEOC is a unique subtype of ovarian neoplasm, which tends to occur in younger women, is confined to the ovaries and has a more indolent natural history. Primary mEOC is unlike metastatic mucinous epithelial cancer, which tends to occur in older women with multiple sites of metastasis (often both ovaries involved) and retains the biological behaviour of the primary tumour [3].

The poor outcome of patients with HGMOC is largely due to two main factors. Firstly, the majority of these patients have incurable advanced stage (stage IV) disease at diagnosis. Secondly, these tumours are largely unresponsive to the ovarian cancer chemotherapy regimen, in particular platinum-based chemotherapy regimen, as first-line and subsequent-line treatment [4]. Historically, mucinous ovarian cancers are treated as a single entity together with epithelial ovarian cancer, as seen in large clinical trials such as ICON3 [5], ICON5 [6] and ICON7 [7].

The distinction between primary and metastatic mucinous adenocarcinoma of the ovary has become a major focus given its importance in predicting outcomes and also to allow appropriate tumour workup and treatment planning. The diagnosis of primary HGMOC and metastatic mucinous epithelial cancer remains challenging although there is now a better recognition by pathologists in distinguishing both subsets of cancer. Advances in imaging techniques and the involvement of multidisciplinary discussions are aiding in differentiating between primary and metastatic mEOC. In a recent retrospective analysis of patients enrolled into the ICON5 trial, where the patients were screened by a panel of experts and treated as ovarian cancer, 68% of stage III and IV HGMOC cases were redefined as metastasis to the surface of ovaries [8]. This was reflected in the poor outcomes of these patients because they had received standard ovarian cancer treatment as part of their adjuvant and palliative treatment. In general, patients with advanced mEOC should be treated as a separate entity requiring an alternative therapeutic approach, such as fluorouracil (5FU) based chemotherapy regimen [9]. Despite strong preliminary support for a change in regimen there is still a universal lack of evidence in directing treatment for this subset of cancer due to the rarity of HGMOC. A recent phase II trial comparing the use of platinum-based chemotherapy versus 5FU-based chemotherapy with or without the use of an anti-angiogenic agent (Bevacizumab) failed due to poor patient accrual. Interestingly, upon specialist pathology review of all cases (n = 36), 52% of mEOC were actually metastatic disease from elsewhere, highlighting again the diagnostic difficulties [10].

The molecular events leading to the development of HGMOC are largely unknown. Gene and protein expression analyses have been performed on well-curated mucinous ovarian cancers to elucidate the key molecular processes allowing a better understanding of the tumour biology and development of biomarkers [11]. In a study published in 2006 by Heinzelmann-Schwarz et al., the gene expression profile of mEOC was distinct, compared with other subtypes of ovarian cancer, in particular, with serous and endometrioid ovarian cancer. mEOC was shown to express genes associated with mucin production and intestinal cell surface adhesion (e.g. LGALS4), demonstrating molecular similarity to malignant intestinal type epithelial cells but with key differences in gene expression, for example, lack of KRAS activity at the transcriptional level [11]. Perhaps surprisingly given earlier reports [12], mutations in p53 are observed in 64% of true primary mEOC [13]. HGMOC were distinguished by having more chromosomal copy number events, although still not as extensively genomically unstable as High Grade Serous Ovarian Cancer (HGSOC) [13].

We describe in our mini-series four of nine consecutive cases who were referred to The Royal Women's Hospital, Melbourne in 2012 and initially treated as primary HGMOC. These cases were annotated with the initial diagnostic work up, surgical procedure and subsequent management, which include follow-up investigations and systemic treatments. We performed RNAseq analysis on fresh frozen tumour samples from four patients who had consented for tumour tissue bio-banking under the Australian Ovarian Cancer Study (AOCS) platform. Within our metastatic HGMOC cohort, we identified one case with a gene and protein expression profile suggestive of a glucagonoma-like NET gastro-intestinal tumour, which was largely unresponsive to 5FU-based chemotherapy. This report highlights the genomic diversity of HGMOC that might account for a variable outcome to treatment and also the potential clinical application of functional genomics in curating a panel of mutation and expression markers to improve diagnostic accuracy.

2. Patients and methods

2.1 Patient selection

The study group consisted of patients referred to and assessed for mEOC at the Department of Gynaecology, Royal Women's Hospital (RWH) in Melbourne, between December 2011 and March 2013. For all patients, the diagnosis of mEOC was confirmed histologically and slides were reviewed by the RWH pathologists.

The Australian Ovarian Cancer Study (AOCS) was approved by Human Research Ethics Committees at the Peter MacCallum Cancer Centre, Queensland Institute of Medical Research, University of Melbourne and all participating hospitals. Additional approval was obtained from the Human Research Ethics Committees at the Royal Women's Hospital and the Walter and Eliza Hall Institute.

Case data were obtained via the CONTRO-engined gemma database, Royal Women's Hospital and the following parameters were collected: histology, age, date of diagnosis, stage of disease, grade, primary surgery (and outcomes), tumour markers (CA-125 and carcinoembryonic antigen) before and after chemotherapy, chemotherapy regimen, clinical outcome of patient following treatments (initial and subsequent lines), and date of death or last follow-up.

HGMOC cases (Grade 2 or 3) were selected for RNAseq analysis based on the availability of fresh frozen tumour sample collected at the time of surgery and patient consent to the AOCS study.

2.2 RNAseq

Fresh frozen tumour tissue was obtained from the bio-bank (AOCS) facility. Total RNA was isolated using the RNeasy kit (Qiagen), and Illumina polyA RNAseq performed according to standard protocols at Australian Genome Research Facility. Libraries were 50 bp single end sequenced in multiplexed pools to an average depth of 50 million reads.

The resulting reads were mapped with Bowtie2 to the human reference genome with local alignment and discarding multi-mapped reads. Reads were summarised to genes using HTSeq and ENSEMBL v69. Differential expression analysis was performed in edgeR [14], comparing the four HGMOC cases as a group (to identify gene expression common to all cases), and each case individually (to allow for high levels of heterogeneity between cases) to a panel of 16 High Grade Serous Ovarian Cancer (HGSOC) cases.

The resulting list of up-regulated genes present in HGMOC was filtered for genes that are expressed in less than 10 anatomical systems in the eGenetics expression resource using ENSEMBL biomart [15].

3. Results

3.1 Patient characteristics

Nine patients with a histologically confirmed diagnosis of high-grade mucinous ovarian cancer presented at the Gynaecology Department of RWH between December 2011 and March 2013 (**Figure 1**). Three patients declined consent to AOCS and were therefore excluded from this study. Of the six patients who consented to AOCS, one did not have fresh frozen tumour tissue stored during the original surgery and another case was excluded due to subsequent diagnosis of pseudomyxoma peritonei. RNAseq analysis was performed on the remaining four cases using tumour tissue snap frozen at surgery. The patients' characteristics were summarised as per **Table 1**. Representative histology images are shown in **Figure 2**.

3.2 Case reports

3.2.1 Tumour 1

Patient #32, a 31-year-old woman with no significant family history of malignancy, presented with a short history of increasing right iliac fossa abdominal pain. She previously had a CT scan 1 month earlier, which showed a large 16 cm complex left ovarian mass. This mass was confirmed by her pre-operative pelvic MRI scan with enlarged para-aortic lymph nodes below the renal artery and no other obvious

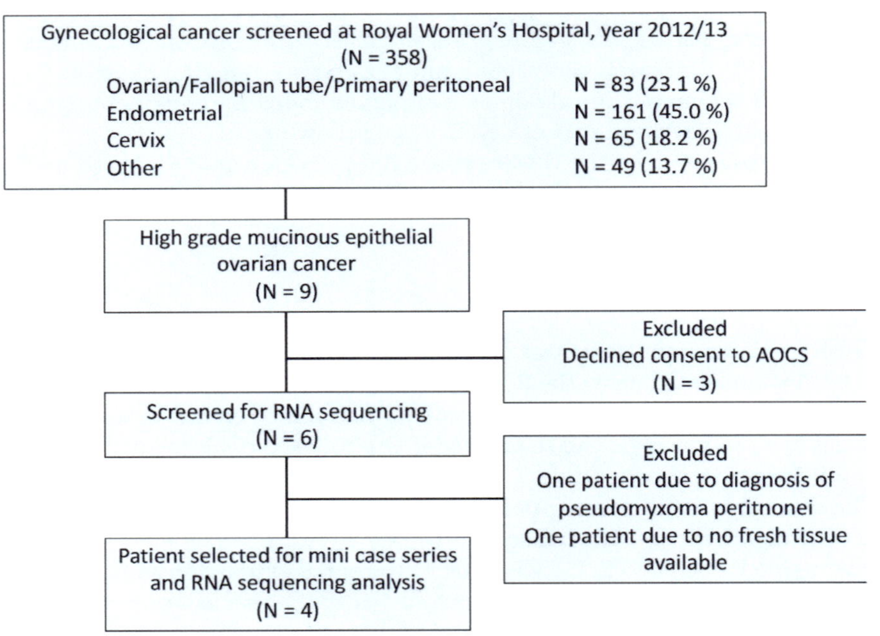

Figure 1.
Patients screened at Royal Women's hospital during 2012/13 being treated as high grade mucinous epithelial ovarian cancer for RNA sequencing analysis.

Patient number	#32	#35	#49	#60
Age (years)	31	34	64	67
Past medical history	Nil	Nil	Non-insulin dependent diabetes mellitus Hypertension Thyroid cyst	Previous metastatic appendix mucinous adenocarcinoama of right ovary (2 years earlier) Oestoarthritis Hypertension
Histopathology				
Histology	Adenocarcinoma with focal intestinal type mucinous differentiation	High-grade adenocarcinoma with focal mucinous differentiation	Mucinous adenocarcinoma with large area of mucin surrounded by signet ring cells - associated with appendiceal tumour with similar histological features	Adenocarcinoma with tumour cells demonstrating focal intracytoplasmic mucin
Immunohistochemistry	CK7, CK19 and CEA diffusely positive, CK20 focally positive	CK7 diffusely strongly positive and CK20 positive in 30-40% of tumour cells, P53 positive in areas of carcinoma	CK20 strongly positive, CK7, WT1 and GCDFP15 negative, Chromogranin and synaptophysin positive	CK20 positive and CK7 negative
Grade	II	III	II	III
Stage	FIGO 1A	FIGO 1C	IV	IV
Laterality	Left	Left	Bilateral	Left
Size	18cm	15cm	7.5cm (right) and 6cm (left)	14cm
Pathologist opinion	May represent primary ovarian carcinoma but need to exclude upper GIT/pancreaobiliary tumour	Consistent with primary HGMOC	Appendiceal primary mucinous adenocarcinoma with neuroendocrine differentiation	Metastatic from previous appendix mucinous adenocarcinoma with similar histopathology features
Baseline tumour markers				
CA125	20	112	6	584
Surgical outcome	Optimal debulk	Optimal debulk	Optimal debulk	Debulking surgery
Post surgery systemic treatment	Nil	Carboplatin and paclitaxel (completed 6 cycles)	5FU-based chemotherapy Radiotherapy - at progression for symptom control	Standard colorectal treatment
Survival outcome	Alive at 5 year follow-up	Alive at 5 year follow-up	Died 4 years later	Lost to follow-up (discharged back to the colorectal team)

Table 1.
Patient characteristics.

lesion identified. This patient underwent total abdominal hysterectomy (TAH), bilateral salpingo-oophorectomy (BSO) and para-aortic lymph node sampling. At surgery, her bowels and intra-peritoneal cavity looked normal. Her tumour histology was reviewed at a multi-disciplinary meeting and was diagnosed as grade 2 primary mEOC stage IA. She received no further systemic treatment. For completion of her cancer assessment, the patient underwent upper gastro-intestinal endoscopy and colonoscopy, which were both normal and subsequently had a PET/CT scan that showed no evidence of metastatic disease. The patient remained alive and well at 5-year follow-up.

3.2.2 Tumour 2

Patient #35 was a 34-year-old woman with no previous significant background medical history and presented to her general practitioner with 1-month history of intermittent lower abdominal pain. Her initial ultra-sound scan organised by her general practitioner showed a large left ovarian cyst and pre-operative MRI scan confirmed a 18 cm complex mixed cystic lesion with a 5 cm solid component associated with moderate ascites. The patient underwent up-front surgery with TAH and BSO. Her peritoneum, abdominal organs and diaphragm appeared to be normal during surgery. The histopathology result confirmed high-grade mucinous adenocarcinoma of the ovary with no surface spread and negative lymph node

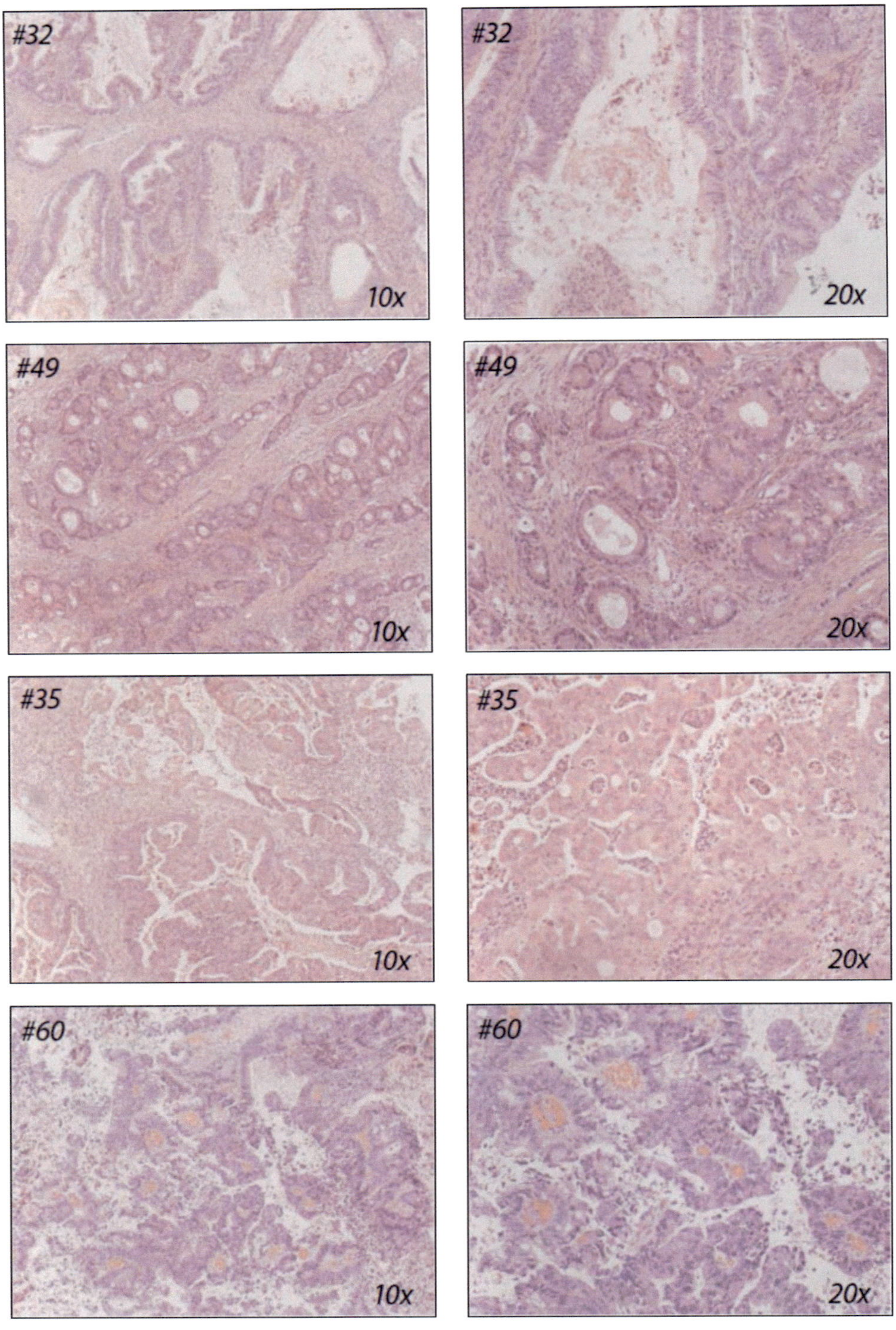

Figure 2.
Histopathology of the four cases: Representative haematoxylin and eosin stained slides presented at 10× and 20× magnification.

involvement. The tumour was stage IC given that the peritoneal washing was positive for malignant cells. Patient received adjuvant ovarian cancer chemotherapy, consisting of carboplatin and paclitaxel, at her local medical oncology centre. She also underwent upper gastro-intestinal endoscopy and colonoscopy as completion of her tumour assessment, which were normal. She remained well and alive at her last follow-up assessment 5 years later.

3.2.3 Tumour 3

Patient #49 was a 64-year-old woman with known type II diabetes mellitus who presented to her local hospital with increasing abdominal pain, nausea, vomiting, and urinary frequency. Her initial CT scan showed a right ovarian mass associated with peritoneal deposits. This was confirmed by her diagnostic laparoscopy that showed a 14 cm ovarian mass adherent to the left adnexa and pouch of Douglas associated with macroscopic tumour deposits on her anterior abdominal wall and omentum. The original biopsy confirmed adenocarcinoma favouring gastro-intestinal tumour. She underwent TAH, BSO, omentectomy and appendectomy. Bilateral ovarian masses were resected during her surgery together with appendiceal and omental nodules. The histopathology confirmed metastatic mucinous adenocarcinoma on both ovaries with evidence of similar tumour effacement of the appendix suggestive of appendiceal origin. It was noted by the pathologist that there was NET differentiation of her mucinous adenocarcinoma with immunohistochemistry staining for chromogranin and synaptophysin positive. She was discharged from hospital following recovery of her surgery to the care of the gastro-intestinal (GI) team. Her case was discussed at the GI tumour board meeting and the expert opinion was to treat this as advanced stage (Stage IV) colorectal cancer with palliative fluorouracil (5FU) based chemotherapy following her surgical debulking procedure. The patient had minimal residual disease prior to commencing her palliative chemotherapy. Her gastroscopy and colonoscopy performed post-operatively showed significant pathology. She completed 8 cycles of FOLFOX (5FU with oxaliplatin) following by single agent 5FU until late 2014. The patient had an interval PET/CT scan performed a year later that showed minimal metabolic activity in known low volume metastatic peritoneal disease. She subsequently presented in 4–6 months later with incomplete bowel obstruction and radiological evidence of slow peritoneal disease progression. Her bowel obstruction resolved with conservative management and she declined further lines of systemic treatment. She received palliative radiation therapy to her peritoneal metastasis with some relief of abdominal symptom. She had multiple admissions to her local hospital in the following 12 months, with bowel-related complications and subsequently passed away in that year, 4 years following the diagnosis of her cancer having only effectively completed one line of systemic treatment.

3.2.4 Tumour 4

Patient #60 was a 67-year-old woman who was diagnosed with metastatic appendiceal mucinous adenocarcinoma of her right ovary 2 years prior to her re-referral with a left ovarian mass. Her initial cancer was treated with surgical removal of the right ovarian and appendiceal mass. Her surgery was complicated with extensive venous thrombo-embolic (VTE) events. She received no systemic treatment following her initial surgery and represented with a 12 cm mixed cystic/solid mass arising from the left ovary based on initial imaging. She underwent second de-bulking surgery following insertion of an inferior vena cava filter for her VTE. This involved the removal of the dense left pelvic tumour mass that was adherent to her bowel, ureter and bladder requiring cystotomy and colostomy. The histopathology report confirmed evidence of adenocarcinoma with focal intracytoplasmic mucin consistent with mucinous adenocarcinoma similar with the original diagnosis 2 years ago. The CK20 was strongly positive and associated with negative staining for CK7. The patient was discharged back to her original colorectal team for further management.

3.3 Transcriptome analysis by RNAseq

Due to the high level of heterogeneity in expression within the HGMOC group, significantly differentially expressed genes were not able to be detected in the group comparison. However, the individual tumour analyses identified a large number of differentially expressed genes. This large number of differentially expressed genes is an expected limitation of this type of analysis, as variance can only be estimated from the control group and there is no suppression of random variability as would be seen in a group of replicates. Because many of these genes were minimally informative, the differentially expressed genes were filtered to identify upregulated genes that are annotated as having organ specific expression and may be informative for the organ of origin. The RNAseq analysis identified 18 genes with a restricted tissue/organ expression pattern that were differentially up regulated in the four tumour samples. These genes were enriched for expression in colon, stomach, pancreas, lung, kidney and skeletal muscle. Only two of the genes, LGALS4 and ERN2, are annotated as expressed in gynaecological tissues and both are also expressed in colonic tissue (**Figure 3**).

3.3.1 Primary mucinous ovarian epithelial carcinoma exhibits a gene expression profile distinct from metastatic mucinous epithelial carcinoma and high-grade serous ovarian cancer

The variable genes identified by transcript profiling revealed that the two primary HGMOC tumours #32 and #35, could be clearly distinguished from the two metastatic mEOC, tumours #49 and #60. A cluster of genes including PGC (encodes a digestive gastric protein), ANAX10 (encodes a calcium- and phospholipid-binding gastric protein), DOUX2 (encodes an oxidase enzyme common in thyroid and GI system) and C12orf36 (non-protein encoding RNA) were up regulated in both tumour #32 and tumour #35. Tumour #49 and tumour #60 had CDH17 (encodes a cadherin superfamily glycoprotein common in gastro-intestinal and pancreatic cells), GUCY2C (encodes for guanylyl cyclase enzyme found in intestinal epithelium) and SCGN (encodes a secretory calcium binding protein in cell cytoplasm) genes up regulated. All four tumours shared in common high expression of seven genes not seen in HGSOC, in particular LGALS4, an intestinal surface cell adhesion molecule that is over-expressed in intestinal carcinomas [16]. LGALS4 had previously been shown to be specifically expressed in mEOC [11]. However, in our cohort, this gene was universally expressed in all four tumours rendering it as a non-distinguishing gene. Interestingly, the two primary HGMOC (tumour #32 and tumour #35) retained some expression of PAX8 and WT1 together with KRT7/CK7 expression as also seen in the HGSOC control panel. The expression of PAX8 in mucinous epithelial ovarian cancer, and the lack of its expression in appendiceal cancers, has been previously described and this further supports the relevance of this gene expression in differentiating the organ of origin of the tumour [17]. With only two mEOC cases this analysis is weakly powered and heavily influenced by the individual cases. Analysis of a larger cohort and validation will be required to identify robust clinical markers.

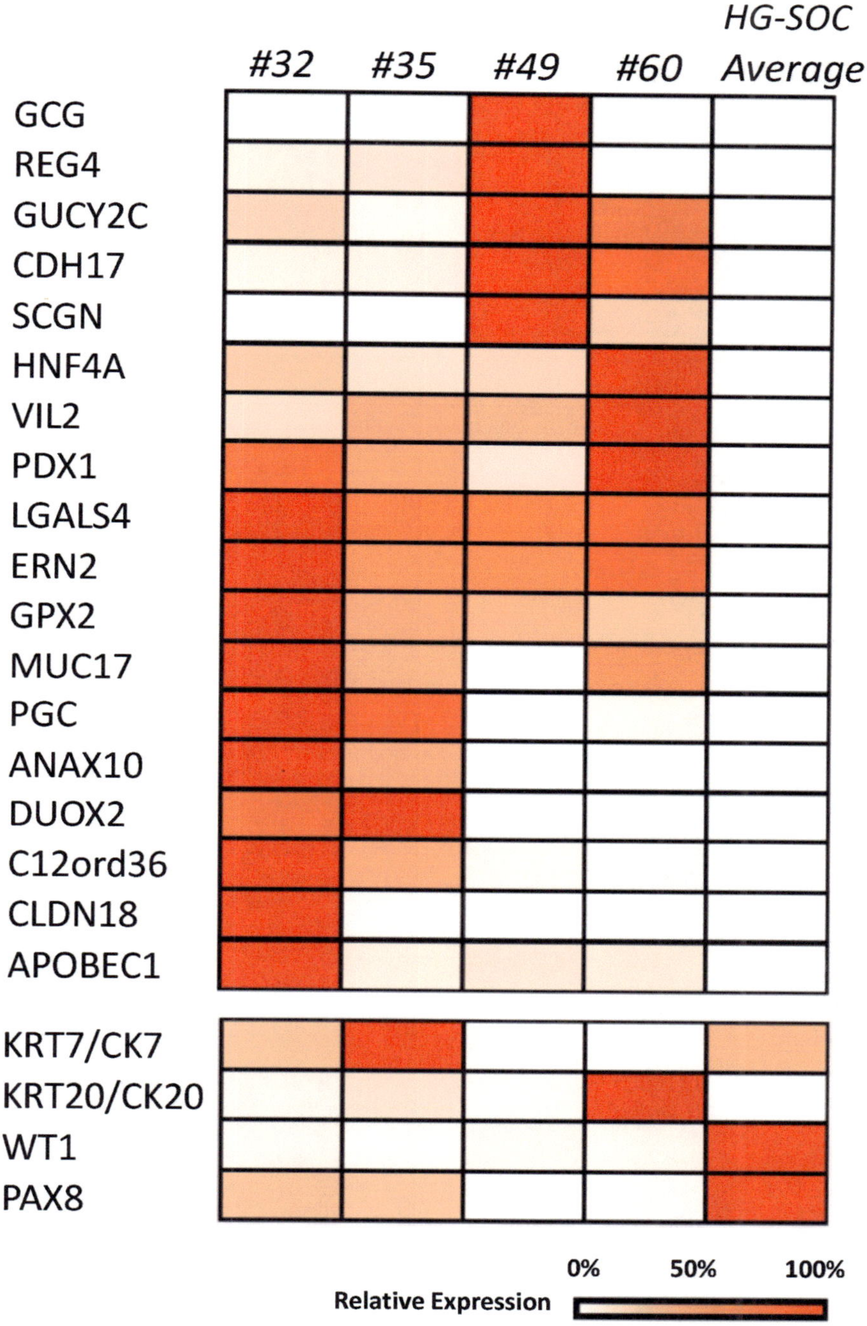

Figure 3.

Heat map of the most differentially expressed genes in the four tumours analysed compared to HGSOC (top panel), and expression comparison of four commonly used markers (lower panel). The tissue specific expression of the listed genes: GCG: pancreas; REGA: GIT (D, Sm, C, R) + appendix; GUCY2C: GIT (D, Sm, C, R); CDH17: GIT (S, D, Sm, C, R) + appendix; SCGN: GIT (S, D, Sm, C, R) + pancreas; HNF4A: GIT (S, D, Sm, C, R) + liver + pancreas + appendix; VIL2: GIT + FGT; PDX1: GIT (D, S) + pancreas; LGALS4: GIT (S, D, S) + gallbladder + appendix; ERN2: GIT (S, D, S, C, R) + appendix; GPX2: GIT + liver + kidney; MUC17: GIT (D, Sm); PGC: S; ANAX10: S; DUOX2: thyroid + stomach; C12ord36: S; CLDN18: S; APOBEC1: Sm; KRT7/CK7: FT. cervix, uterine, liver, gallbladder, pancreas; KRT20/CK20: GIT (D, S, C, R); WT1: FGT; PAX8: FGT. GIT: gastro-intestinal tract; D: duodenum; S: stomach; Sm: small intestine; C: caecum; R: rectum; FGT: female genital tract; FT; fallopian tube.

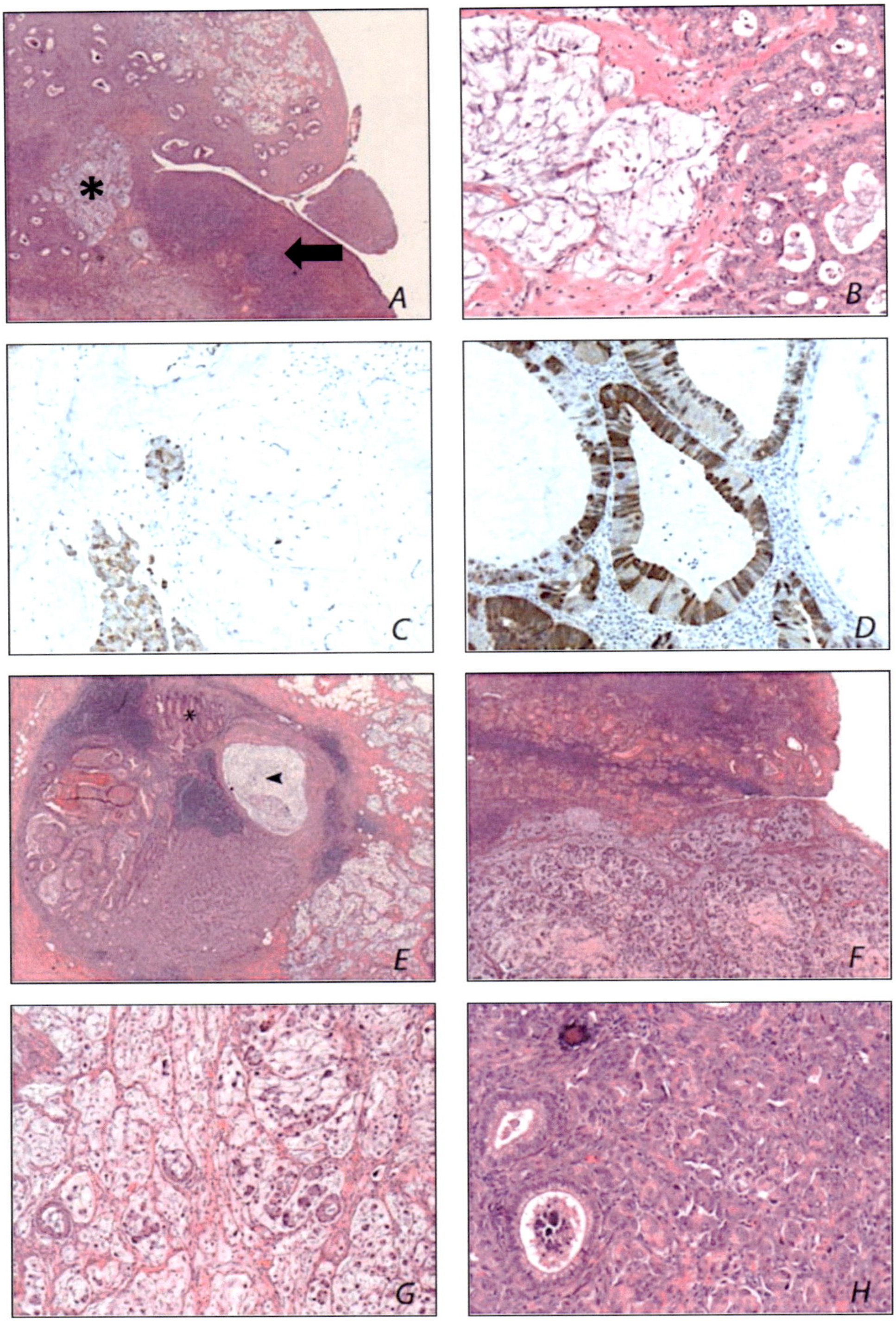

Figure 4.
A. Adenocarcinoma seeding in the ovary; normal ovarian tissue (arrow), mucinous glandular component of adenocarcinoma (*); prominent stromal desmoplasia can be typically seen in tumours that secondarily involve the ovary (5× magnification); B. Adenocarcinoma in the ovary (20× magnification); C. Chromogranin immunohistochemical staining shows strong and diffuse reactivity (20× magnification); D. Glucagon immunohistochemical staining shows strong reactivity in tumour cells (20× magnification); E. Adenocarcinoma infiltrating the appendix (5× magnification); lumen of appendix (arrow); adenocarcinoma (*); F. Adenocarcinoma in the appendix (20× magnification); G. Adenocarcinoma in the appendix (20× magnification); H. Adenocarcinoma in the appendix (20× magnification).

3.3.2 Identification of tumour #49 as a glucagonoma-like neuroendocrine tumour of likely appendiceal origin by transcriptome analysis

The RNAseq analysis identified up regulation of GCG, a gene that encodes for glucagon, in tumour #49. GCG accounted for ~5% of transcriptional output indicating a high level of glucagon expression. The original histopathology report on the resected tumour confirmed evidence of NET differentiation within the mucinous adenocarcinoma, with positive IHC staining for chromogranin and synaptophysin. Our findings were returned to the original pathologist at RWH and further IHC for glucagon protein expression was performed. Strong glucagon staining was seen in the tumour cells by IHC, confirming the RNAseq findings (**Figure 4**). This "glucagonoma"-like tumour may have either a pancreatic origin or may have originated from the appendix as clinically implicated (**Figure 4**).

This patient's case was discussed at the GI tumour board meeting, and despite the finding of our RNAseq analysis, it was treated as a standard colorectal cancer given the rarity of NET differentiated mucinous adenocarcinoma of the appendix. It was difficult to ascertain the full effect of CRC/5FU-based chemotherapy regimen on this patient given the limited line of treatment received and perceived minimal residual disease post-surgery. Unfortunately, the patient declined further chemotherapy at first progression but survived for a further 2 years receiving only palliative radiation treatment to problematic intra-abdominal lesions.

4. Discussion

True mucinous epithelial ovarian carcinomas are a rare subtype of ovarian cancer. In our limited case cohort, half of the mEOC seen in our institute at a given period of time were re-diagnosed as metastatic mucinous epithelial carcinoma. This posed a challenge for both the pathologists and surgical team to provide an accurate and timely diagnosis of the cancer and enable the delivery of optimal treatment. Clinical and radiological information, such as patient age, laterality of tumour, tumour stage and to some extent tumour marker CA125 can guide diagnosis prior surgery [3]. Ultimately, it is the histology of the resected tumour that allows accurate assessment of tumour origin based on the pattern of protein expression seen by IHC and morphology [8]. However, in patient #60 case, a previous history of appendiceal tumour should have raised the suspicious for metastatic recurrence of the tumour.

Our pilot RNAseq study indicated that tumours initially diagnosed as mEOC can be a diverse collection of disease, and that gene expression analysis has the potential to identify prognostically useful subsets. Categorising based on gene expression and identifying genetic aberrations is likely to greatly assist in selection of the optimal treatment for each individual patient. While RNAseq for each individual patient is an impractical method for tumour identification, the observations from this study contributed to the design of a larger study, GAMuT—Genomic Analysis of Mucinous Tumours, which will compare HGMOC to low grade and borderline cases to identify prognostic and therapeutically useful gene expression signatures (Australian National Health and Medical Research (NH&MRC) Funded Study—APP1045783). This study will allow the selection of a panel of mutation and expression markers to elucidate the tumour organ of origin, thus providing some guidance in treatment selection.

We highlighted the identification of a very rare "glucagonoma-like" NET appendiceal tumour in our series of mEOC to indicate the reliability of functional genomics in identifying rare conditions. This diagnosis is in context with the patient's clinical findings and also with IHC proving glucagon protein expression only apparent after the RNA sequencing results were available. In hindsight, it is hard to predict if this patient would have benefited from repeated surgical resection of recurrent tumour [18], or to NET based treatment regimens, such as mTOR inhibition (everolimus) [19] or multiple tyrosine kinase inhibitor (sunitinib, pazopanib) [20, 21]. Furthermore, the patient did not exhibit glucagon syndrome and her glucagon serum level was never tested. Nevertheless, clinically tumour #49 behaved like a NET tumour with slow indolent progression and localised complication. Unfortunately, in this case, the problematic tumour caused repeated bowel obstructive symptoms requiring multiple hospital admissions in the months leading up to the patient's death.

The recognition of diversity of tumour subtypes even within a rare tumour population is important especially in designing clinical trials. Given the small number of patients available for accruement, it is vital that we accurately stratify patients into treatment arms and identify robust biomarkers early. A very rare tumour within a rare tumour subtype can pose a challenging issue in terms of being an outlier that would skew the outcome in a clinical trial and also in optimising treatment for this patient based on available evidence (which is lacking). These issues will need to be addressed in any clinical trials pertaining to rare cancer.

Acknowledgements

We thank Margot Osinski (Royal Women's Hospital) for database assistance and AOCS: The Australian Ovarian Cancer Study Group was supported by the U.S. Army Medical Research and Materiel Command under DAMD17-01-1-0729. The AOCS also acknowledges the cooperation of the participating institutions in Australia and acknowledges the contribution of the study nurses, research assistants and all clinical and scientific collaborators to the study. The complete AOCS Study Group can be found at www.aocstudy.org. We would like to thank the women who participated in these research programs.

Author details

Gwo Yaw Ho[1,2,3,4,7*], Sumitra Ananda[1,3,4,8], Cassandra J. Vandenberg[1,4], Orla McNally[7], Jeanne Tie[1,3,4], Kylie Gorringe[3,4], David Bowtell[3], Jan Pyman[7], Matthew J. Wakefield[1,4] and Clare L. Scott[1,3,4,5,6,7]

1 Walter and Eliza Hall Institute, Parkville, Australia

2 Monash University, Melbourne, Australia

3 Peter MacCallum Cancer Centre, Melbourne, Australia

4 The University of Melbourne, Melbourne, Australia

5 Royal Melbourne Hospital, Parkville, Australia

6 Monash Medical Centre, Clayton, Australia

7 Royal Women's Hospital, Parkville, Australia

8 Western Health, Melbourne, Australia

*Address all correspondence to: ho.g@wehi.edu.au

References

[1] Schiavone MB et al. Natural history and outcome of mucinous carcinoma of the ovary. American Journal of Obstetrics and Gynecology. 2011;**205**:480.e1-480.e8

[2] Perren TJ. Mucinous epithelial ovarian carcinoma. Annals of Oncology. 2016;**27**:i53-i57

[3] Khunamornpong S et al. Primary and metastatic mucinous adenocarcinomas of the ovary: Evaluation of the diagnostic approach using tumor size and laterality. Gynecologic Oncology. 2006;**101**:152-157

[4] Pignata S et al. Activity of chemotherapy in mucinous epithelial ovarian cancer: A retrospective study. BMC Cancer. 2008;**8**:252

[5] Investigators, I.T. Paclitaxel plus carboplatin versus standard chemotherapy with either single-agent carboplatin or cyclophosphamide, doxorubicin, and cisplatin in women with ovarian cancer: The ICON3 randomised trial. The Lancet. 2002;**360**:505-515

[6] Bookman MA. GOG0182-ICON5: 5-arm phase III randomized trial of paclitaxel (P) and carboplatin (C) vs combinations with gemcitabine (G), PEG-liposomal doxorubicin (D), or topotecan (T) in patients (pts) with advanced-stage epithelial ovarian (EOC) or primary peritoneal (PPC) carcinoma. Journal of Clinical Oncology. 2006:**24**(18_suppl):5002-5002. DOI: 10.1200/jco.2006.24.18_suppl.5002

[7] Oza AM et al. Standard chemotherapy with or without bevacizumab for women with newly diagnosed ovarian cancer (ICON7): Overall survival results of a phase 3 randomised trial. Lancet Oncology. 2015;**16**:928-936

[8] Zaino RJ et al. Advanced stage mucinous adenocarcinoma of the ovary is both rare and highly lethal. Cancer. 2010;**117**:554-562

[9] Hess V. Mucinous epithelial ovarian cancer: A separate entity requiring specific treatment. Journal of Clinical Oncology. 2004;**22**:1040-1044

[10] Gore ME et al. Multicentre trial of carboplatin/paclitaxel versus oxaliplatin/capecitabine, each with/without bevacizumab, as first line chemotherapy for patients with mucinous epithelial ovarian cancer (mEOC). Journal of Clinical Oncology. 2015. DOI: 10.1200/jco.2015.33.15_suppl.5528

[11] Heinzelmann-Schwarz VA et al. A distinct molecular profile associated with mucinous epithelial ovarian cancer. 2006:1-10. DOI: 10.1038/sj.bjc.6603003

[12] Shih I-M, Kurman RJ. Ovarian tumorigenesis. The American Journal of Pathology. 2010;**164**:1511-1518

[13] Cheasley D et al. The molecular origin and taxonomy of mucinous ovarian carcinoma. Nature Communications. 2019:1-11. DOI: 10.1038/s41467-019-11862-x

[14] Robinson MD, McCarthy DJ, Smyth GK. edgeR: A bioconductor package for differential expression analysis of digital gene expression data. Bioinformatics. 2009;**26**:139-140

[15] Magali R et al. Ensembl core software resources: Storage and programmatic access for DNA sequence and genome annotation. Database. 2017:1-11. DOI: 10.1093/database

[16] Grotzinger C et al. LI-cadherin: A marker of gastric metaplasia and neoplasia. Gut. 2001;**49**:78-81

[17] Laury A et al. A comprehensive analysis of PAX8 expression in human epithelial tumors. The American Journal of Pathology. 2011;**35**:816

[18] Al-Faouri A, Ajarma K, Alghazawi S, Al-Rawabdeh S, Zayadeen A. Case report glucagonoma and glucagonoma syndrome: A case report with review of recent advances in management. Case Reports in Surgery. 2016:1-3. DOI: 10.1155/2016/1484089

[19] Yao JC et al. Everolimus for the treatment of advanced, non-functional neuroendocrine tumours of the lung or gastrointestinal tract (RADIANT-4): A randomised, placebo-controlled, phase 3 study. The Lancet. 2016;**387**:968-977

[20] Dahan L et al. Sunitinib malate for the treatment of pancreatic neuroendocrine tumors. New England Journal of Medicine. 2011;**364**:501-513

[21] Grande E et al. Pazopanib in pretreated advanced neuroendocrine tumors: A phase II, open-label trial of the Spanish task force Group for Neuroendocrine Tumors (GETNE). Annals of Oncology. 2015;**26**:1987-1993

Chapter 4

Therapeutic Effect of Glypican-3 Gene Silencing Using siRNA for Ovarian Cancer in a Murine Peritoneal Dissemination Model

Mai Hazekawa, Takuya Nishinakagawa, Tomoyo Kawakubo-Yasukochi and Manabu Nakashima

Abstract

Ovarian cancer is known to be the most lethal gynecologic cancer. It has been reported that Glypican-3 (Gpc3) expression induces immune responses, promotes the progression in ovarian cancer. Then, we focused on this Gpc3 gene silencing, tried to prepare siRNA delivery system. In this chapter, we introduce one of the therapeutic proposals in terms of novel drug delivery system using siRNA as a targeting medicine. This chapter introduces our works about preparation of siRNA-PLGA hybrid micelles to deliver the siRNA into the ovarian cancer cells and to evaluate gene silencing effects in mice model. As a result, siRNA-PLGA hybrid micelles were shown to effectively inhibit Gpc3 expression *in vitro*. In addition, siRNA-PLGA hybrid micelles also decreased the number of tumor nodes in the mesentery *in vivo*. These results suggested that Gpc3 could be a target molecule for ovarian cancer treatment and siRNA-PLGA hybrid micelles could be an effective siRNA delivery tool even *in vivo*.

Keywords: siRNA, ovarian, Glypican-3, micelle, PLGA

1. Introduction

Epithelial ovarian carcinoma (EOC) is the most lethal gynecological malignancy. EOC accounts for about 90% of all ovarian cancers and distributed over the most common histotypes: high-grade serous (HGSC, 70%), low-grade serous (LGSC, < 5%), endometrioid (EC, 10%), mucinous (MC, 3–4%) and clear cell ovarian carcinoma (CCC, 10%) [1]. Five-year survival rates differ significantly across the histotypes, with drastically lower survival rates for serous carcinoma (SC (HGSC and LGSC), 43%) compared with EC (82%), MC (71%) and CCC (66%) in the USA. CCC is a comparatively rare tumor, depending on the geographic location. In west countries, OCCC represents <10% of all EOC. In contrast, the incidence of CCC

IntechOpen

was reportedly 25% of EOC in Japan. The high number of patients (80%) with SC is diagnosed at advanced stages (stages III and IV). While, CCC which has the second number of patients (25%) after SC, is predominantly diagnosed at stage I (65%) [2]. Thus, CCC has different character compared with SC. Five-year survival rate at stage I for SC and CCC is same (80%). While, five-year survival rate at stage IV for SC is 40% and stage I of CCC is 25%. CCC has a very poor prognosis. One of the reasons is that CCC is associated with greater chemoresistance and a poorer prognosis compared with other EOC subtypes. Particularly for recurrent CCC, the response rate (RR) to salvage chemotherapy was extremely low. Previous studies have indicated that high L-type amino acid transporter 1 (LAT1), which belongs to system L, a Na^+-independent carrier that transports large neutral amino acids, expression was associated with poorer prognosis and chemoresistance in CCC [3]. Furthermore, hepatocyte nuclear factor 1β (HNF1β) and glutaminolysis contribute for the chemoresistance to platinum-based antineoplastic agents of CCC through the intrinsically increased glutathione (GSH) bioavailability [4]. Therefore, novel and innovative strategies are required to improve outcomes for patients with CCC that is refractory to chemotherapy.

Glypican-3 (GPC3) is a member of the glypican family of heparan sulfate proteoglycans. GPC3 regulates cell proliferation signals by binding growth factors such as Wnt, fibroblast growth factor, and insulin-like growth factor and plays an important role in the proliferation and differentiation of embryonic cells [5–7]. GPC3 is expressed in various fetal tissues (liver, lung, kidney, and placenta) but is not detected in normal postnatal tissue due to DNA methylation-induced epigenetic silencing [8, 9]. While, previous studies showed that GPC3 was overexpressed in several malignant tumors, including hepatocellular carcinoma (HCC), CCC and melanoma. Particularly, GPC3 is detected in ≥80% of patients with HCC caused by hepatitis B or C [10, 11]. The function of membrane-anchored GPC3 in these cancers is unknown, but it is likely involved in the neoplastic transformation of HCC [12]. Membrane-bound GPC3 can be cleaved and secreted into the blood. Mammalian GPC family members are cleaved at GPI anchor level by endogenous GPI phospholipase D [13]. Thus, various forms of GPC3 protein are present in blood, although their functions remain unclear. Given these features, GPC3 is useful not only as a target for cancer immunotherapy but also as a novel tumor marker.

Small interfering or silencing RNA (siRNA) technologies are based on the inhibition of gene expression or translation by siRNAs targeting messenger RNA selectively [14]. Gene interference therapy using siRNA has great potential for treatment of wide variety of diseases [15], ranging from cancer [16–19] to viral infection [20, 21] and brain disorder [22, 23]. The benefit of applying this technology to cancer therapy is that siRNA can target genes which are specific for tumor cells, leaving healthy, non-tumor tissue unaffected. Despite their medical potential, the clinical translation of siRNA technologies has up to now been limited. This limited progress is due to the difficulties of delivering siRNA *in vivo*. Unprotected siRNAs are easily degraded in the bloodstream, and siRNAs alone do not translocate across cell membrane [24]. In addition, it has been reported that siRNAs can be immunogenic [25]. Therefore, safe and efficient carriers must be developed for siRNA delivery to protect siRNA from nuclease action and at the same time triggers intracellular uptake *in vivo* [26, 27].

In our previous study, we prepared slow release formulation using biodegradable polymer (poly(lactide-co-glycolide), PLGA) such as micro-/nano particles [28]. Recently, we engaged to prepare the siRNA delivery system using PLGA for anti-metastasis therapy.

In this chapter, we report the therapeutic effect of Gpc3 gene silencing in ovarian cancer, and introduce the finding about a novel siRNA delivery system of micelles for nucleic acid therapy based on our data [29].

2. Effect of anti-metastasis in ovarian cancer caused by Glypican-3 gene silencing

2.1 Role of Grypican-3 in ovarian cancer

GPC3, 55–65 kDa protein consisting of 580 amino acids, is a heparan sulfate chain proteoglycan (HSPGs) bound to cell membrane by a glycosylphosphatidylinositol (GPI) anchor. This protein is expressed in the liver and kidney of healthy fetuses but is hardly expressed in adults, except in the placenta. Loss of function mutations of GPC3 leads to Simpson-Golabi-Behmel syndrome (SGBS), a rare X-linked disorder (X chromosome, Xq26) with significant overgrowth [5], which has also been observed in GPC3-null mice [30] because the gene shows high homology between humans and mice. GPC3 is expressed ubiquitously in the embryo but is reduced in the central nervous system (CNS) in adults [31]. Thus, GPC3 is considered to be one of the factors affecting prenatal development and metabolism originally. On the other hand, GPC3 is especially overexpressed in HCC [10, 11], CCC [32, 33], melanoma [34], and lung cancer [35]. Although the precious function of GPC3 remains unclear, it has been strongly suggested that it is related to the malignant transformation, accelerating cell growth and increasing inflammatory reaction [36].

The Wnt/Frizzled/β-catenin pathway is activated in about 50% of HCCs. Wt3a has been shown to mediate the GPC3-induced growth of HCCs via the canonical Wnt/β-catenin pathway [6, 37]. Sulfated heparan sulfate glycosaminoglycan (HSGAG) chains of GPC3 and other HSPGs are potential substrates for desulfation at the 6-O position by human sulfate 2 (SULF2). It has been reported that SULF2 activates Wnt/β-catenin signaling in HCC cells, and this process is GPC3-dependent and can be independent of exogenous Wnts [38]. In a previous study, a human monoclonal antibody against GPC3 inhibited Wnt3a/β-catenin signaling in HCC cells and antitumor activity *in vivo* [39]. Furthermore, blocking the heparan sulfate chains on GPC3 with human monoclonal antibody against GPC3 also reduced c-Met activation in hepatocyte growth factor (HGF)-treated HCC cells and 3D-cultured spheroids. GPC3 is involved in HCC cell migration and motility through HS chain-mediated cooperation with the HGF/Met pathway [40].

Although the role of GPC3 in HCC has been reported little by little, the role of GPC3 in ovarian cancer, especially CCC expressed GPC3, has been remained unclear. So recurrent or persistent CCC has been reported as having a potentially chemoresistant phenotype against conventional cytotoxic agents, leading to poorer prognosis. Thus, novel treatment approaches must be adopted for CCC. With compelling evidence that EOC is an immunogenic tumor, immunotherapeutic approaches are currently being evaluated and should be optimized based on histology-specific features. Previous research also suggested that GPC3 peptide vaccinations may hold a significant impact to prolong survival of patients with refractory CCC, allowing them to maintain quality of life with no serious toxicities [41].

Based on these, we focused on knocking down of GPC3 gene therapy for ovarian cancer using siRNA which can be expected to be effective in clinical practice. Then, we evaluated the efficiency of siRNA-PLGA hybrid micelles targeted to Gpc3 on ovarian cancer *in vitro* and examined its antitumor effects *in vivo* in a mouse peritoneal dissemination model.

2.2 Effect of anti-metastasis caused by knocking down of Grypican-3 using LPEI coating siRNA-PLGA hybrid micelles *in vivo*

The synthesis of siRNA-PLGA hybrid was described briefly as follows. PLGA was activated by DCC and NHS. Activated PLGA reacted with 3-(2-pyridyldithio) propionyl hydrazide (PDPH) as a cross-linker. After PDPH activated, PLGA (PLGA-PDPH) was used for siRNA conjugation. A thiol-modified double-strand siRNA was reacted with PLGA-PDPH, siRNA-PLGA hybrid was synthesized via a disulfide exchange reaction. The synthesized siRNA-PLGA hybrid conjugates spontaneously formed self-assembled micelles in aqueous solutions, resulting to form micelle with siRNA side facing the outer shell as shown in **Figure 1A** and **C**. Furthermore, we also prepared liner polyethylenimine (LPEI)-coated siRNA-PLGA micelles, its surface was positive charged by cationic polymer, to increase the efficiency of intracellular uptake as shown in **Figure 1D**.

Measurement of critical micelle concentration (**Figure 2**) and distribution of particle (**Figure 3**) were performed to evaluate the physical properties of micelles. The mean diameter and zeta potential of siRNA-PLGA hybrid micelles were about 110 nm and about −40 mV, respectively. The zeta potentials of siRNA-PLGA hybrid micelle were changed from negative charge to positive charge by LPEI coating.

Until now, the best agents for siRNA delivery are cationic lipids and polycations, i.e. polyelectrolytes bearing multiple positive charges to increase intracellular uptake *in vivo* [42, 43]. From these previous data, LPEI coating micelle can be expected its clinical potential *in vivo* because positive charge caused by LPEI makes micelles easy to be taken into the cell.

The GPC3 levels in HM-1 cell line, which is mouse ovarian cancer cell line, treated with siRNA-PLGA hybrid micelles were then evaluated by western blotting.

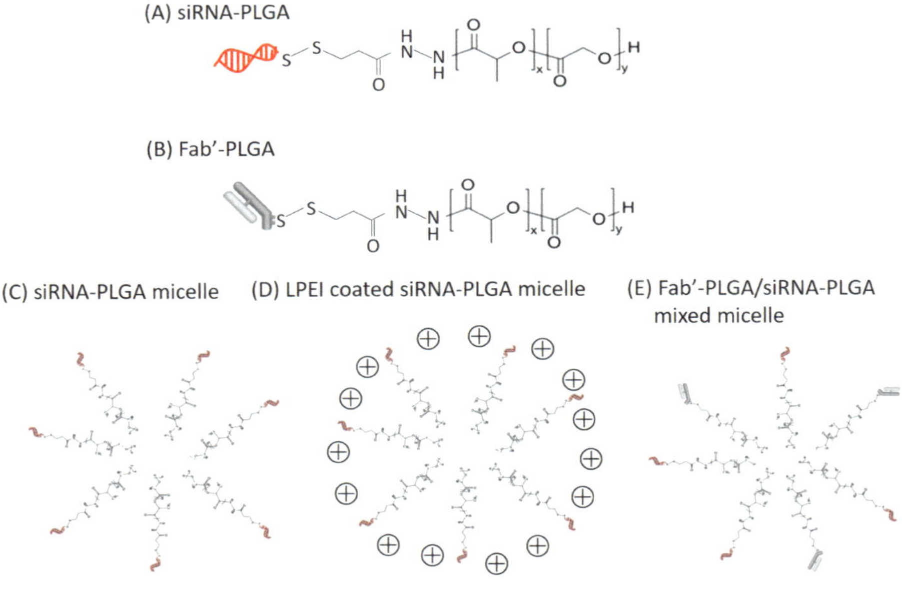

Figure 1.
(A) and (B) Structure of siRNA-PLGA hybrid and Fab'-PLGA hybrid via a cleavable disulfide linkage. (C)–(E) Schematic diagram for siRNA-PLGA hybrid micelle structure in an aqueous environment.

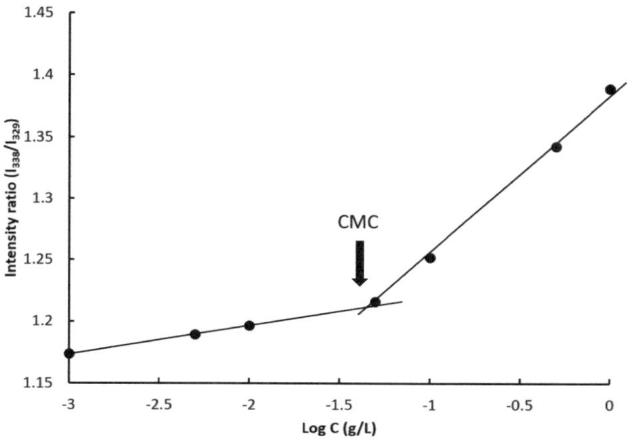

Figure 2.
Critical micelle concentration (CMC) detected by measuring the relative excitation intensity ratio of pyrene at emission of 329 nm and 338 nm (I_{338}/I_{329}).

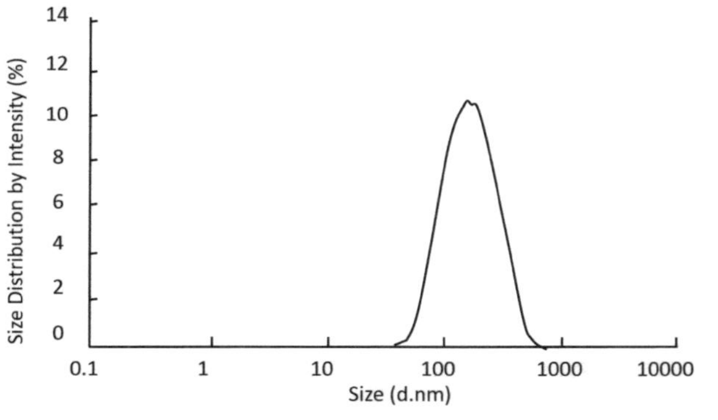

Figure 3.
Size distribution of siRNA-PLGA hybrid micelles.

As shown in **Figure 4**, siRNA-PLGA hybrid micelles significantly suppressed GPC3 expression compared with the control.

Assessment of antitumor effects of these micelles in a murine peritoneal dissemination model was performed by intraperitoneal (i.p.) injection as topical treatment. In general, topical administration is often more effective because it is easy to react since the medicine is close to the disease lesion [44]. The number of disseminated nodules and the peritoneal fluid volumes were evaluated at 15 days after injection of the HM-1 cells. As shown in **Figure 5**, the number of disseminated nodules and the volume of peritoneal fluid siRNA-PLGA hybrid micelle-treated groups were significantly low compared with the control. Next, GPC3 levels in the cell lysates of peritoneal cells collected from the peritoneal fluid were evaluated by western blotting.

As shown in **Figure 6**, the levels of IFN-γ, IL-6, and TNF-α in mice treated with uncoated and LPEI-coated siRNA-PLGA hybrid micelles were significantly suppressed compared with the control. GPC3 expression in the lymphocytes such as B cells, T cells and macrophages in the peritoneal fluid of mice, was detected by western blotting. From these results, there is a possibility that the therapeutic effect was induced by GPC3 gene knockdown of not only cancer cell but also lymphocytes in the peritoneal fluid as the additive effects.

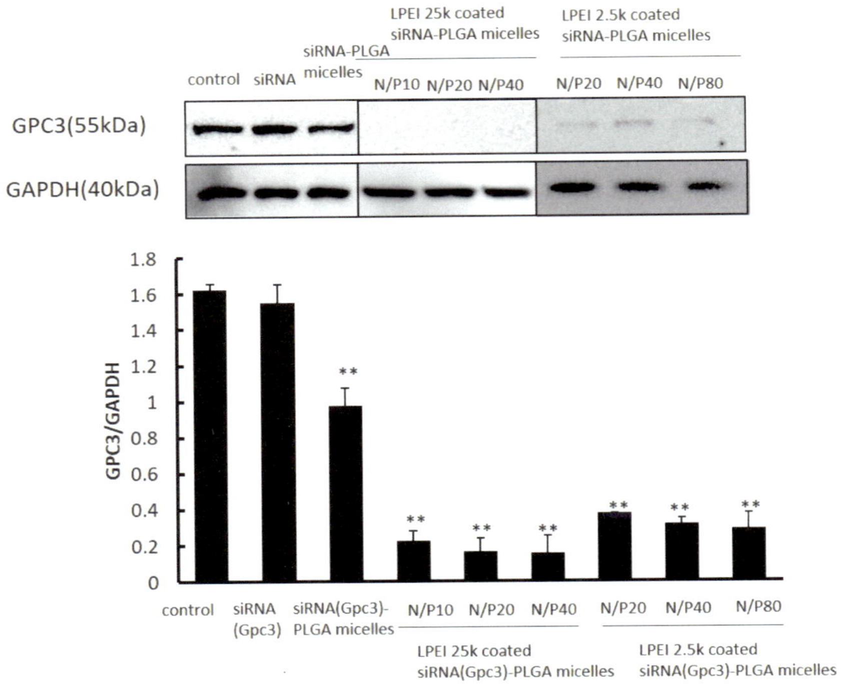

Figure 4.
Western blot analysis of GPC3levels in HM-1 cells treated with siRNA-PLGA hybrid micelles in vitro. *Data represent the mean ± SD (n = 3). **p < 0.01 versus the control group (Bonferroni test/ANOVA). Cited from Ref. [29]. Reprinted with permission from Elsevier.*

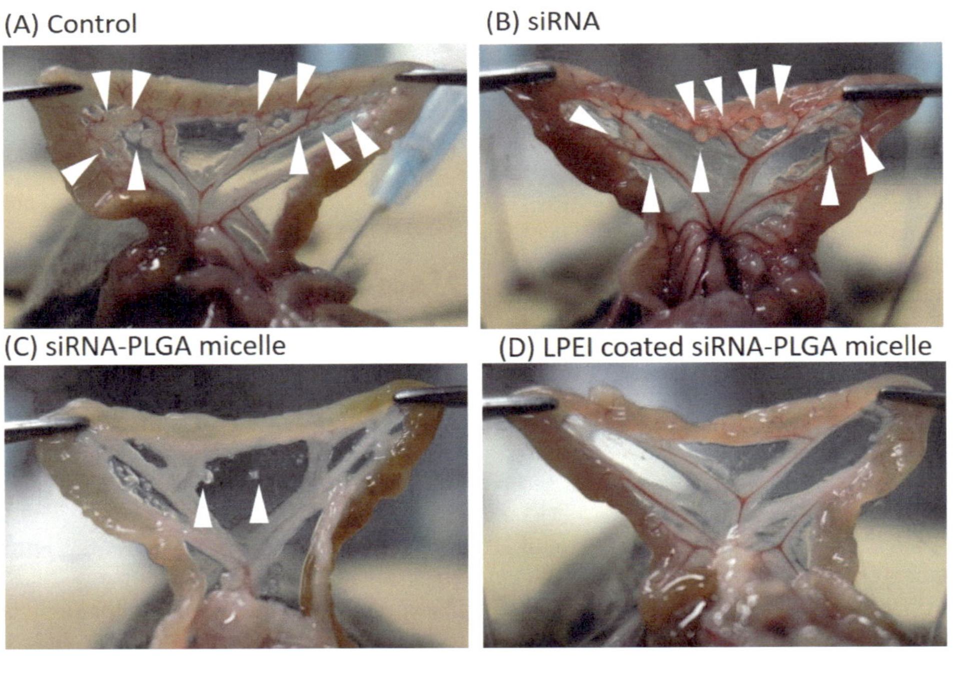

Figure 5.
Anti-metastasis effects of siRNA-PLGA micelles in a mouse peritoneal dissemination model. Representative images of the mesentery after laparotomy. Cited from Ref. [29]. Reprinted with permission from Elsevier.

2.3 Recognition of cancer cell using Fab′-PLGA/siRNA-PLGA hybrid mixed micelle *in vitro*

In previous study, we reported that Gpc3 knocking down using siRNA-PLGA hybrid micelle by intraperitoneal injection was effective to suppress the metastasis in peritoneal dissemination of ovarian cancer mice model [29]. However, it is

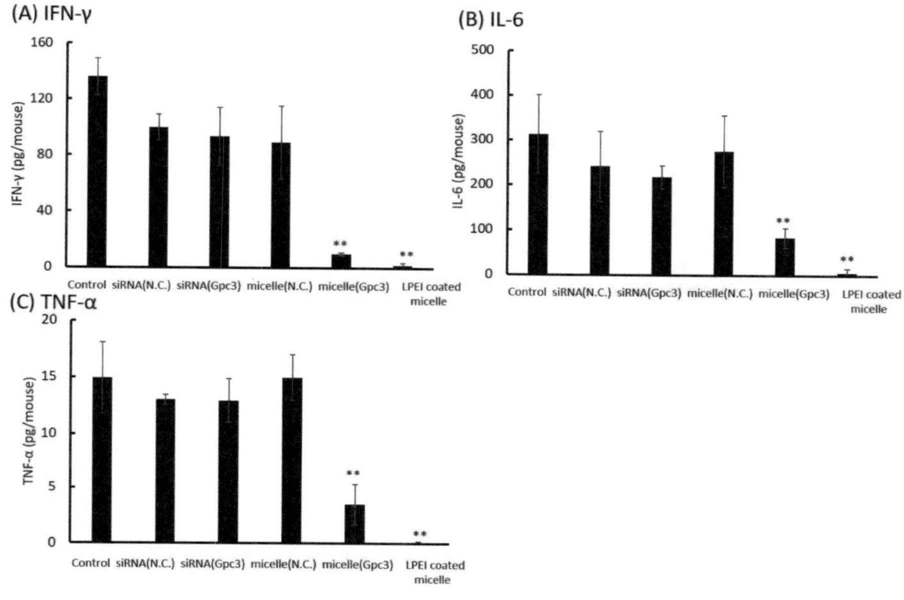

Figure 6.
*Effect of GPC3 knockdown caused by treatment with siRNA-PLGA micelles on the secretion of IFN-γ, IL-6, TNF-α in the peritoneal fluid in a mouse peritoneal dissemination model. Data represent the mean ± SD (n = 5). **p < 0.01 versus the control group (Bonferroni test/ANOVA). Cited from Ref. [29]. Reprinted with permission from Elsevier.*

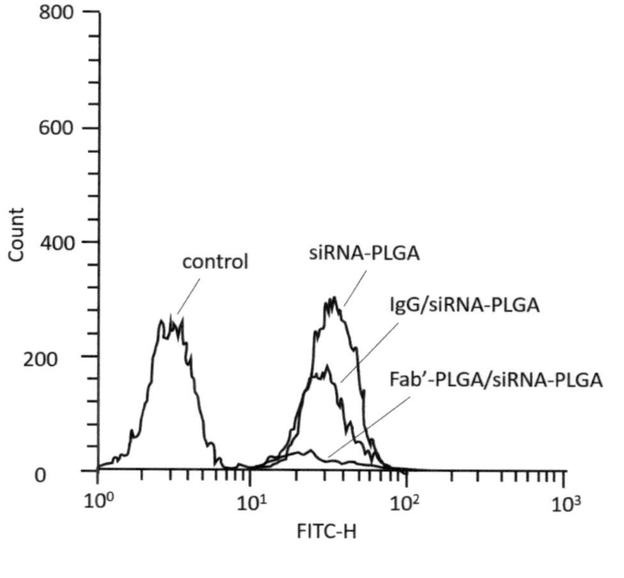

Figure 7.
Efficiency of intracellular uptake of Fab′-PLGA/–Alexa 488 labeling siRNA-PLGA hybrid mixed micelles in vitro by flow cytometry analysis.

necessary to develop a carrier which is "targeting" and "systemically administable". That is why, we prepared Fab′-PLGA/siRNA-PLGA mixed micelle to recognize the target cell. Fab′-PLGA hybrid was synthesized in a same method as siRNA-PLGA hybrid was synthesized. The drug design was described in **Figure 1B** and **E**.

As shown in **Figure 7**, *in vitro* experiment, intracellular uptake of siRNA using Fab′-PLGA/siRNA-PLGA mixed micelle was significantly increased compared with control. In particular, cytotoxicity was accelerated caused by treatment with Fab′-PLGA/siRNA-PLGA mixed micelle compared with siRNA-PLGA hybrid micelle. This result suggests that the characteristics of the targeting used by antibody may be expected to have an additive effect of the function of Fab′ itself in addition to the increase in the intracellular uptake efficiency by cell recognition. In some antibodies, the target protein knockdown effect is dramatically obtained using Fab′-PLGA/siRNA-PLGA mixed micelle (data not shown). From these results, Fab′-PLGA/siRNA-PLGA mixed micelles are believed to be useful as one of the targeting formulations to recognize the target cell.

3. Expected side effect caused by gene therapy and limitation of assessment using animal

3.1 Off-target effects caused by RNAi

The technique of RNAi in the medical field is expected to have not only therapeutic effects for human induced by knock-down specific genes but also suffers from off-target effects. Previous study reported that algorithm or open-source desktop software was developed to design RNAi sequences to exert strong and selective suppression of target genes and predict off-target [45, 46]. However, it is difficult to predict specific side effects that appear due to off-target effects in human. Furthermore, we suggested that the details of the off-target effect are often unclear due to the fact that commercial nucleic acid medications have a short period of use. In some cases, mouse results may not be compatible with humans because off-target effects vary by its sequences though there were no noticeable side effects in our experiment *in vivo*.

3.2 Cytotoxicity of exogenous siRNA or polymer in development of formulation

Until now, some polyplex or lipoplex with high membrane permeability formulations have been used for siRNA delivery system [47, 48]. A number of polymers have been popularly utilized to form stable and nanocomplexes with its cytotoxicity problem [27, 49–53]. PEI is also probably the most frequently used polycation in gene delivery, our LPEI-coated micelles did not exhibit cytotoxic effects. The fact that no toxicity was found in our experiments at the concentrations we used was consist with previous reports [54]. The greatest feature of this micelle is that it consists of a safe polymer, PLGA. PLGA is known as one of the biodegradable polymers used in marketed medication [55]. In some cases, siRNA can be immunogenic such as virus vectors induce multiple component of the immune response, cytotoxic T-lymphocyte (CTL) response can be elicited against viral gene products of exogenous transgene products [25]. Regarding the immunogenicity of this micelle, it is unlikely that immunogenicity was shown due to the fact that cytokines in the peritoneal fluid were suppressed.

3.3 Limitation of assessment using animal

In the future as a next step, immunodeficient mice would be indispensable when we establish human model such as patient-derived xenograft (PDX) model. However, there is possibility that we cannot comprehend whether the micelle has medical potential when immunodeficient mice are used because GPC3 might be a molecule that is strongly associated with the immune system. That is why, we considered that we should further examine the usefulness of this therapy using micelles for human cancer cells based on our data using murine cell because there are different characteristics between murine and human cancer cells.

4. Conclusion

In conclusion, our results could indicate that Gpc3 gene silencing using siRNA has a possibility as an effective new therapeutic approach without side effects in ovarian cancer, especially CCC with GPC3 expression. Furthermore, this GPC3 targeting gene therapy is also useful for high GPC3 expression cancer such as HCC, melanoma and lung cancer if appropriate carrier is developed to deliver siRNA to target cancer cell by i.v. in the future.

In addition, this finding is the first study to show that siRNA-PLGA hybrid micelles can effectively deliver siRNA to cancer cells *in vivo* at a low dose with significant anti-metastatic effect on murine ovarian cancer. We expect that novel formulation with more specific effects like siRNA including drug delivery system would be developed for malignant ovarian cancer therapy in the future.

Acknowledgements

This work was supported by JSPS KAKENHI Grant Number JP17K08477, Fukuoka Foundation for Sound Health Cancer Research Fund, and funds (No. 181045) from the Central Research Institute of Fukuoka University.

Conflict of interest

The authors declare no conflict of interest.

Author details

Mai Hazekawa*, Takuya Nishinakagawa, Tomoyo Kawakubo-Yasukochi and Manabu Nakashima
Department of Immunological and Molecular Pharmacology, Faculty of Pharmaceutical Sciences, Fukuoka University, Fukuoka, Japan

*Address all correspondence to: mhaze@fukuoka-u.ac.jp

References

[1] Engqvist H, Parris TZ, Kovács A, Nemes S, Werner Rönnerman E, De Lara S, et al. Immunohistochemical validation of COL3A1, GPR158 and PITHD1 as prognostic biomarkers in early-stage ovarian carcinomas. BMC Cancer. 2019;**19**(1):928. DOI: 10.1186/s12885-019-6084-4

[2] Torre LA, Trabert B, DeSantis CE, Miller KD, Samimi G, Runowicz CD, et al. Ovarian cancer statistics, 2018. CA: A Cancer Journal for Clinicians. 2018; **68**(4):284-296. DOI: 10.3322/caac.21456

[3] Sato K, Miyamoto M, Takano M, Furuya K, Tsuda H. Significant relationship between the LAT1 expression pattern and chemoresistance in ovarian clear cell carcinoma. Virchows Archiv. 2019;**474**(6):701-710. DOI: 10.1007/s00428-019-02520-0

[4] Lopes-Coelho F, Gouveia-Fernandes S, Gonçalves LG, Nunes C, Faustino I, Silva F, et al. HNF1β drives glutathione (GSH) synthesis underlying intrinsic carboplatin resistance of ovarian clear cell carcinoma (OCCC). Tumour Biology. 2016;**37**(4):4813-4829. DOI: 10.1007/s13277-015-4290-5

[5] Pilia G, Hughes-Benzie RM, MacKenzie A, Baybayan P, Chen EY, Huber R, et al. Mutations in GPC3, a glypican gene, cause the Simpson-Golabi-Behmel overgrowth syndrome. Nature Genetics. 1996;**12**(3):241-247. DOI: 10.1038/ng0396-241

[6] Capurro MI, Xiang YY, Lobe C, Filmus J. Glypican-3 promotes the growth of hepatocellular carcinoma by stimulating canonical Wnt signaling. Cancer Research. 2005;**65**(14): 6245-6254. DOI: 10.1158/0008-5472.CAN-04-4244

[7] Gutiérrez J, Brandan E. A novel mechanism of sequestering fibroblast growth factor 2 by glypican in lipid rafts, allowing skeletal muscle differentiation. Molecular and Cellular Biology. 2010;**30**(7):1634-1649. DOI: 10.1128/MCB.01164-09

[8] Lin H, Huber R, Schlessinger D, Morin PJ. Frequent silencing of the GPC3 gene in ovarian cancer cell lines. Cancer Research. 1999;**59**(4):807-810

[9] Nakatsura T, Nishimura Y. Usefulness of the novel oncofetal antigen glypican-3 for diagnosis of hepatocellular carcinoma and melanoma. BioDrugs. 2005;**19**(2):71-77. DOI: 10.2165/00063030-200519020-00001

[10] Nakatsura T, Yoshitake Y, Senju S, Monji M, Komori H, Motomura Y, et al. Glypican-3, overexpressed specifically in human hepatocellular carcinoma, is a novel tumor marker. Biochemical and Biophysical Research Communications. 2003;**306**(1):16-25. DOI: 10.1016/s0006-291x(03)00908-2

[11] Capurro M, Wanless IR, Sherman M, Deboer G, Shi W, Miyoshi E, et al. Glypican-3: A novel serum and histochemical marker for hepatocellular carcinoma. Gastroenterology. 2003;**125**(1):89-97. DOI: 10.1016/s0016-5085(03)00689-9

[12] Shirakawa H, Suzuki H, Shimomura M, Kojima M, Gotohda N, Takahashi S, et al. Glypican-3 expression is correlated with poor prognosis in hepatocellular carcinoma. Cancer Science. 2009;**100**(8): 1403-1407. DOI: 10.1111/j.1349-7006.2009.01206.x.

[13] Metz CN, Brunner G, Choi-Muira NH, Nguyen H, Gabrilove J, Caras IW, et al. Release of GPI-anchored membrane proteins by a cell-associated GPI-specific phospholipase D. The EMBO Journal. 1994;**13**(7):1741-1751

[14] Whitehead KA, Langer R, Anderson DG. Knocking down barriers: Advances in siRNA delivery. Nature Reviews. Drug Discovery. 2009;**8**: 129-138. DOI: 10.1038/nrd2742

[15] Wittrup A, Lieberman J. Knocking down disease: A progress report on siRNA therapeutics. Nature Reviews. Genetics. 2015;**16**:543-552. DOI: 10.1038/nrg3978

[16] Kim HJ, Kim A, Miyata K, Kataoka K. Recent progress in development of siRNA delivery vehicles for cancer therapy. Advanced Drug Delivery Reviews. 2016;**104**:61-77. DOI: 10.1016/j.addr.2016.06.011

[17] Oh YK, Park TG. siRNA delivery systems for cancer treatment. Advanced Drug Delivery Reviews. 2009;**61**: 850-862. DOI: 10.1016/j.addr.2009.04.018

[18] Lei Y, Tang L, Xie Y, Xianyu Y, Zhang L, Wang P, et al. Gold nanoclusters-assisted delivery of NGF siRNA for effective treatment of pancreatic cancer. Nature Communications. 2017;**8**:1-15. DOI: 10.1038/ncomms15130

[19] Lee H, Kim IK, Park TG. Intracellular trafficking and unpacking of sirna/quantum dot-pei complexes modified with and without cell penetrating peptide: Confocal and flow cytometric fret analysis. Bioconjugate Chemistry. 2010;**21**:289-295. DOI: 10.1021/bc900342p

[20] Morrissey DV, Lockridge JA, Shaw L, Blanchard K, Jensen K, Breen W, et al. Potent and persistent in vivo anti-HBV activity of chemically modified siRNAs. Nature Biotechnology. 2005;**23**:1002-1007. DOI: 10.1038/nbt1122

[21] Gu J, Al-Bayati K, Ho EA. Development of antibody-modified chitosan nanoparticles for the targeted delivery of siRNA across the blood-brain barrier as a strategy for inhibiting HIV replication in astrocytes. Drug Delivery and Translational Research. 2017;**7**: 497-506. DOI: 10.1007/s13346-017-0368-5

[22] Kuwahara H, Nishina K, Yoshida K, Nishina T, Yamamoto M, Saito Y, et al. Efficient in vivo delivery of siRNA into brain capillary endothelial cells along with endogenous lipoprotein. Molecular Therapy. 2011;**19**:2213-2221. DOI: 10.1038/mt.2011.186

[23] Zheng M, Tao W, Zou Y, Farokhzad OC, Shi B. Nanotechnology-based strategies for siRNA brain delivery for disease therapy. Trends in Biotechnology. 2018;**36**:562-575. DOI: 10.1016/j.tibtech.2018.01.006

[24] Wang J, Lu Z, Wientjes MG, Au JL. Delivery of siRNA therapeutics: Barriers and carriers. The AAPS Journal. 2010;**12**: 492-503. DOI: 10.1208/s12248-010-9210-4

[25] Thomas CE, Ehrhardt A, Kay MA. Progress and problems with the use of viral vectors for gene therapy. Nature Reviews. Genetics. 2003;**4**:346-358. DOI: 10.1038/nrg1066

[26] Dominska M, Dykxhoorn DM. Breaking down the barriers: siRNA delivery and endosome escape. Journal of Cell Science. 2010;**123**:1183-1189. DOI: 10.1242/jcs.066399

[27] Gary DJ, Puri N, Won YY. Polymer-based siRNA delivery: Perspectives on the fundamental and phenomenological distinctions from polymer-based DNA delivery. Journal of Controlled Release. 2007;**121**:64-73. DOI: 10.1016/j.jconrel.2007.05.021

[28] Hazekawa M, Kojima H, Haraguchi T, Yoshida M, Uchida T. Effect of self-healing encapsulation on the initial burst release from PLGA microspheres containing a long-acting

prostacyclin agonist, ONO-1301. Chemical & Pharmaceutical Bulletin. 2017;**65**(7):653-659. DOI: 10.1248/cpb.c17-00025

[29] Hazekawa M, Nishinakagawa T, Kawakubo-Yasukochi T, Nakashima M. Glypican-3 gene silencing for ovarian cancer using siRNA-PLGA hybrid micelles in a murine peritoneal dissemination model. Journal of Pharmacological Sciences. 2019;**139**(3): 231-239. DOI: 10.1016/j.jphs.2019.01.009

[30] Cano-Gauci DF, Song HH, Yang H, McKerlie C, Choo B, Shi W, et al. Glypican-3-deficient mice exhibit developmental overgrowth and some of the abnormalities typical of Simpson-Golabi-Behmel syndrome. The Journal of Cell Biology. 1999;**146**(1):255-264. DOI: 10.1083/jcb.146.1.255

[31] Fransson LA. Glypicans. The International Journal of Biochemistry & Cell Biology. 2003;**35**(2):125-129. DOI: 10.1016/s1357-2725(02)00095-x

[32] Stadlmann S, Gueth U, Baumhoer D, Moch H, Terracciano L, Singer G. Glypican-3 expression in primary and recurrent ovarian carcinomas. International Journal of Gynecological Pathology. 2007;**26**(3): 341-344. DOI: 10.1097/pgp.0b013e31802d692c

[33] Maeda D, Ota S, Takazawa Y, Aburatani H, Nakagawa S, Yano T, et al. Glypican-3 expression in clear cell adenocarcinoma of the ovary. Modern Pathology. 2009;**22**(6):324-832. DOI: 10.1038/modpathol.2009.40

[34] Nakatsuka T, Kageshita T, Ito S, Wakamatsu K, Monji M, Ikuta Y, et al. Identification of glypican-3 as a novel tumor marker for melanoma. Clinical Cancer Research. 2004;**10**(19): 6612-6621. DOI: 10.1158/1078-0432.CCR-04-0348

[35] Lin Q, Xiong LW, Pan XF, Gen JF, Bao GL, Sha HF, et al. Expression of GPC3 protein and its significance in lung squamous cell carcinoma. Medical Oncology. 2012;**29**(2):663-669. DOI: 10.1007/s12032-011-9973-1

[36] Luo C, Shibata K, Suzuki S, Kajiyama H, Senga T, Koya Y, et al. GPC3 expression in mouse ovarian cancer induces GPC3-specific T cell-mediated immune response through M1 macrophages and suppresses tumor growth. Oncology Reports. 2014;**32**(3): 913-921. DOI: 10.3892/or.2014.3300

[37] Capurro MI, Shi W, Sandal S, Filmus J. Processing by convertases is not required for glypican-3-induced stimulation of hepatocellular carcinoma growth. The Journal of Biological Chemistry. 2005;**280**(50):41201-41206. DOI: 10.1074/jbc.M507004200

[38] Lai JP, Oseini AM, Moser CD, Yu C, Elsawa SF, Hu C, et al. The oncogenic effect of sulfatase 2 in human hepatocellular carcinoma is mediated in part by glypican 3-dependent Wnt activation. Hepatology. 2010;**52**(5): 1680-1689. DOI: 10.1002/hep.23848

[39] Gao W, Kim H, Feng M, Phung Y, Xavier CP, Rubin JS, et al. Inactivation of Wnt signaling by a human antibody that recognaizes the heparan sulfate chains of glypican-3 for liver cancer therapy. Hepatology. 2014;**60**(2): 576-587. DOI: 10.1002/hep.26996

[40] Gao W, Kim H, Ho M. Human monoclonal antibody targeting the heparan chains of glypican-3 inhibits HGF-mediated migration and motility of hepatocellular carcinoma cells. PLoS One. 2015;**10**(9):e0137664. DOI: 10.1371/journal.pone.0137664

[41] Suzuki S, Sakata J, Utsumi F, Sekiya R, Kajiyama H, Shibata K, et al. Efficacy of glypican-3-derived peptide vaccine therapy on the survival of patients with refractory ovarian clear

cell carcinoma. Oncoimmunology. 2016; **5**(11):e1238542. DOI: 10.1080/2162402X.2016.1238542

[42] Khurana B, Goyal AK, Budhiraja A, Arora D, Vyas SP. siRNA delivery using nanocarriers—An efficient tool for gene silencing. Current Gene Therapy. 2010; **10**:139-155. DOI: 10.2174/156652310791111010

[43] Vader P, van der Aa LJ, Storm G, Schiffelers RM, Engbersen JF. Polymeric carrier systems for siRNA delivery. Current Topics in Medicinal Chemistry. 2012;**12**:108-119. DOI: 10.2174/156802612798919123

[44] Dakwer GR, Zagato E, Delanghe J, Hobel S, Aigner A, Denys H, et al. Colloidal stability of nano-sized particles in the peritoneal fluid: Towards optimizing drug delivery systems for intraperitoneal therapy. Acta Biomaterialia. 2014;**10**(7):2965-2975. DOI: 10.1016/j.actbio.2014.03.012

[45] Tiuryn J, Szczurek E. Learning signaling networks from combinatorial perturbations by exploiting siRNA off-target effects. Bioinformatics. 2019; **35**(14):i605-i614. DOI: 10.1093/bioinformatics/btz334

[46] Lück S, Kreszies T, Strickert M, Schweizer P, Kuhlmann M, Douchkov D. siRNA-finder (si-fi) software for RNAi-target design and off-target prediction. Frontiers in Plant Science. 2019;**10**:1023. DOI: 10.3389/fpls.2019.01023

[47] Hunter AC. Molecular hurdles in polyfectin design and mechanistic background to polycation induced cytotoxicity. Advanced Drug Delivery Reviews. 2006;**58**:1523-1531. DOI: 10.1016/j.addr.2006.09.008

[48] Lv H, Zhang S, Wang B, Cui S, Yan J. Toxicity of cationic lipids and cationic polymers in gene delivery. Journal of Controlled Release. 2006;**114**: 100-109. DOI: 10.1016/j.jconrel.2006.04.014

[49] Hagerman PJ. Flexibility of RNA. Annual Review of Biophysics and Biomolecular Structure. 1997;**26**: 139-156. DOI: 10.1146/annurev.biophys.26.1.139

[50] Kebbekus P, Drasper DE, Hagerman P. Persistence length of RNA. Biochemistry. 1995;**34**:4354-4357. DOI: 10.1021/bi00013a026

[51] Shah SA, Brunger AT. The 1.8 A crystal structure of a statically disordered 17 base-pair RNA duplex: Principles of RNA crystal packing and its effect on nucleic acid structure. Journal of Molecular Biology. 1999;**285**: 1577-1588. DOI: 10.1006/jmbi.1998.2385

[52] Spaqnou S, Miller AD, Keller M. Lipidic carriers of siRNA: Differences in the formulation, cellular uptake, and delivery with plasmid DNA. Biochemistry. 2004;**43**:13348-13356. DOI: 10.1021/bi048950a

[53] Pavan GM, Albertazzi L, Danani A. Ability to adapt: Different generations of PAMAM dendrimers show different behaviors in binding siRNA. The Journal of Physical Chemistry. B. 2010;**114**: 2667-2675. DOI: 10.1021/jp100271w

[54] Mok H, Lee SH, Park JW, Park TG. Multimeric small interfering ribonucleic acid for highly efficient sequence-specific gene silencing. Nature Materials. 2010;**9**(3):272-278. DOI: 10.1038/nmat2626

[55] Okada H. One- and three-month erlease injectable microspheres of LH-RH superagonist leuprorelin acetate. Advanced Drug Delivery Reviews. 1997; **28**(1):43-70

Section 2

Updates in Radiation Therapy in Gynaecological Malignancies

Chapter 5

Dosimetric and Radiobiological Evaluation of Combined Radiotherapy of Cervical Cancer Based on the VMAT Technique

Evgeniia Sergeevna Sukhikh and Leonid Grigorievich Sukhikh

Abstract

A dosimetric and radiobiological investigation of the possibility to replace the traditional combined radiation therapy (3D-CRT + high-dose-rate brachytherapy (HDR-BT)) of cervical cancer with the following combinations, ^{60}Co + VMAT, 3D-CRT + VMAT, and VMAT + VMAT, without change of total course dose and the number of fractions is described. For the investigation, the data of 11 patients with a diagnosis of cervical cancer (stages $T_{2b}N_xM_0$ and $T_3N_xM_0$) who received a course of combined radiotherapy was used. The 3D-CRT + high-dose-rate brachytherapy (HDR-BT) combination of dose delivery techniques was used as the basic one. The following fractionation regimes for combined radiotherapy were simulated: external beam radiation therapy (RT) (EBRT) of the first stage, total dose 50 Gy and fractional dose 2 Gy (25 fractions), and the second stage—total dose 28 Gy and fractional dose 7 Gy (4 fractions). Total combined RT course dose amounted to EQD_2 = 89.7 Gy. Simulation results show that there is a technical possibility of replacing the second stage of combined RT of cervical cancer by EBRT based on the VMAT technique. Implementation of the VMAT technique allows increasing the uniformity of irradiated volume coverage compared with traditional high-dose rate. While using the VMAT technique, the tolerant levels of organs at risk are not exceeded.

Keywords: intracavitary brachytherapy, external beam radiation therapy, cervical cancer, intensity-modulated radiotherapy, combined radiotherapy

1. Introduction

In the treatment of cervical cancer, the main methods include surgical treatment, chemotherapy, and radiation therapy (RT), which can be used either separately or in combination with each other [1–3]. The combination of two consecutive stages of irradiation with different dose delivery techniques, i.e., external beam radiotherapy (EBRT) and intracavitary high-dose-rate brachytherapy, is called combined RT [1–6]. At the first stage of combined RT, the clinical tumor volume and regional lymph nodes are irradiated in total doses up to 44–50 Gy with fraction dose equal to 2 Gy depending on the widespread nature of the process. At the second stage of the combined RT, the clinical tumor volume is irradiated in the mode of dose boost when the dose per fraction is increased to 6–7.5 Gy delivered in 4 or 5 fractions resulting in the total dose equal to 28–30 Gy. The goal of the total combined RT course is to achieve a total EQD_2 dose equal to 90 Gy delivered to the clinical tumor volume in less than 50 days of treatment [2–7].

From the point of view of dose delivery technologies, the first stage of combined RT is EBRT based on one of the methods: conventional RT, 3D conformal RT (3D-CRT), or methods with intensity-modulated radiation (IMRT and VMAT) [8, 9]. The photon radiation sources used are gamma apparatus with ^{60}Co sources and photon energy of 1.25 MeV or linear electron accelerators (linacs) with a photon energy equal to 6 or 10 MeV. When using conventional irradiation with gamma apparatus, there are difficulties in creating a conformal dose field that reduces the dose loads on critical organs, and, consequently, it is hard to improve the uniformity of coverage with a dose of the target volume; therefore, this technique, at present, is not very popular. However, from the point of view of operation and maintenance, the gamma apparatus is simpler and more convenient than linacs. According to IAEA, there are 240 gamma apparatuses in Russia and only 197 linacs. For comparison, in Germany, there are 523 linacs and only 20 gamma apparatuses [10]. From this point of view, the development of techniques for the best possible use of gamma apparatuses is an important task for Russia and other developing countries.

The second stage of combined RT is usually implemented using intracavitary HDR-BT based on gamma-emitting radionuclides ^{60}Co or ^{192}Ir [2–7]. The advantages of BT are the possibility of delivering a high dose to a clinical tumor volume with a relatively low dose load on OARs (bladder and rectum). Most of the radiotherapy departments in Russia are equipped with equipment that allows performing BT in HDR mode. However, BT has several significant drawbacks compared with EBRT. The main one is the substantial heterogeneity of the coverage of the clinical target volume, where doses in the range from 90 to 300% of the prescribed dose are delivered. BT is also a less comfortable procedure for patients because they experience painful sensations when inserting implants into the uterine cavity, which requires anesthesia. Dosimetric planning of BT needs conduction of topographic preparation using CT or magnetic resonance tomography (MRI) with implants inserted followed by a tight vaginal tamponade, to prevent their possible displacement inside the patient during transportation to the treatment table [2, 3, 5]. Optimization of the dose distribution in BT can be regulated only by introducing sectoral blocks into a Manchester (Fletcher)-type applicator (nozzle with an intrauterine endostat) or additional needles for interstitial implantation, which is even more complicated and requires anesthetic management. On the other hand, with BT, no additional margin from the clinical tumor volume (CTV) is required, which should consider the inaccuracy of dose delivery from fraction to fraction, i.e., creating a planned target volume (PTV), which is mandatory for EBRT. Because irradiation occurs from the inside, and not from the outside, in the case of movement of the organ with the implant inserted, the implant will move along with the organ [2–6].

The development of EBRT technologies has led to the widespread implementation of IMRT and VMAT dose delivery techniques, which allow delivery of single doses of up to 7 Gy to a target without exceeding tolerant levels for OARs. The VMAT method with large dose fractions is widely used, for example, in the treatment of prostate carcinomas [11–22]. The first investigations devoted to the study of the possibility of replacing BT with EBRT during the second stage of combined RT started in 2012 [18]. The goal of such investigations was to change BT with EBRT in hypofractionation mode for patients for whom BT was not possible for various reasons.

The aim of this work was to carry out a dosimetric and radiobiological planning of the replacement of traditional combined radiation therapy (3D-CRT + HDR BT) by combinations of ^{60}Co + VMAT, 3D-CRT + VMAT, and VMAT + VMAT while preserving the value of the total dose delivered and the number of fractions. The paper presents a comparison of radiation loads on tumor volumes and critical organs using different combinations of irradiation at the first and second stages, namely, 3D-CRT + HDR BT, conventional RT ^{60}Co + VMAT, 3D-CRT + VMAT, and VMAT + VMAT. The study was conducted using tomographic data of 11 patients with cervical cancer.

2. Combined radiotherapy

Anatomical data of 11 patients with cervical cancer (squamous carcinoma) stages $T_{2b}N_0M_0$ (six patients) and $T_3N_0M_0$ (five patients) were used for investigation. The patients received no surgery due to the fact that for stages T_2 and T_3, the surgery is not the best treatment [13]. The patients were selected randomly between the patients who have received combined radiotherapy for half a year at Tomsk Regional Oncology Center. Patients' age was in the range from 55 to 57 years. All patients had received courses of standard combined radiotherapy using EBRT with 3D-CRT (Elekta Synergy linac, 10 MeV, AB Elekta) or conventional radiotherapy based on ^{60}Co (Theratron Equinox 100) followed by HDR BT (Multisource HDR, Bebig). The prescribed total dose for EBRT amounted to 50 Gy given in 25 fractions (2 Gy/fr). During the HDR BT, the total dose amounted to 28 Gy given in 4 fractions (7 Gy/fr). The total course dose assuming $\frac{a}{b} = 10$ Gy for the tumor was equal to BED = 107.6 Gy and EQD_2 = 89.7 Gy, which agreed with Refs. [2–7]. All patients received concomitant cisplatin chemotherapy weekly.

Different irradiation techniques were compared for dosimetric investigation. During the first stage of combined radiotherapy, we used conventional RT with ^{60}Co, 3D-CRT using 10 MeV photons, and VMAT technique with 10 MeV photons. The second stage modalities included either HDR BT or VMAT with 10 MeV photons. The total dose values, as well as the fractionation regimen, were the same as during irradiation.

The OARs included bladder and rectum. The irradiation constraints are listed in **Table 1**. During the study, we assumed that $\frac{\alpha}{\beta} = 8$ Gy for the bladder and $\frac{\alpha}{\beta} = 3.9$ Gy for the rectum [11]. The data were taken from the QUANTEC protocols [23, 24], RTOG 0415 [25], GYN GES ESTRO [4], and other recommendations.

Organ at risk	QUANTEC [12, 13]	RTOG 0415 [14]	EBRT+BT
Rectum	$V_{50} < 50\%$ $V_{60} < 35\%$ $V_{65} < 25\%$ $V_{70} < 20\%$ $V_{75} < 15\%$	$V_{59} < 50\%$ $V_{64} < 35\%$ $V_{69} < 25\%$ $V_{74} < 15\%$	$D_{2cc} < 75$Gy [3, 15] $D_{2cc} < 70$Gy [2, 4]
Bladder	$V_{65} < 50\%$ $V_{70} < 35\%$ $V_{75} < 25\%$ $V_{80} < 15\%$	$V_{64} < 50\%$ $V_{69} < 35\%$ $V_{74} < 25\%$ $V_{79} < 15\%$	$D_{2cc} < 90$Gy [2–4, 15]

Table 1.
The tolerant levels of critical organs for all radiotherapy courses which include EBRT and BT or only the EBRT for two stages based on QUANTEC [23, 24], RTOG 0415 [25], GYN GES ESTRO [4], and other recommendations [26].

The data in **Table 1** are presented as $V_x < y\%$, which means that the organ volume equal to y% of the total volume should not receive a dose greater than x Gy EQD_2. Late third-grade radiation reactions are possible for the bladder if each of these levels is exceeded. For the rectum, second-grade (<15%) and third-grade reactions (<10%) are possible if the levels are exceeded [23, 24]. The data presented in **Table 1** for EBRT are taken from the statistics of radiation complications obtained during the treatment of prostate carcinomas. Because EBRT is widely used to treat this disease, we used these data, while we found no data for EBRT used along with treatment of cervical cancer due to the extremely rare use of EBRT for the second stage of combined radiotherapy.

2.1 The first-stage EBRT

Patient data for the first stage EBRT were obtained using the CT Toshiba Aquilion (Toshiba, Japan). The scanning step was equal to 3 mm. Patients were in the supine position due to the better immobilization possible [2–5]. A contrast substance was used during topometric preparation for the better identification of structures of interest: vessels, involved lymph nodes, tumor, bowel, bladder, and vagina. The rectosigmoid and the bladder were treated according to international recommendations [2–5] to minimize internal motion and ensure reproducibility during dose planning and treatment.

Because of the use of CT, only the CTV-T included the whole uterus. The PTV-T safety margin was approximately equal to 10 mm to ensure full coverage of the CTV during treatment course [2–5].

The pelvic lymph node (CTV-N) region included parametrial, para-rectal, internal iliac, external iliac, presacral, and iliaca communis. PTV-N included CTV-N plus an additional 10 mm margin. In the case of anatomical barriers such as the bone or uninvolved muscle/fascia, a smaller margin value was used [2–5].

PTV-T and PTV-N were joined to PTV-TN, and the prescription was defined for PTV-TN as follows: $D95 \geq V95\%$ and $D107 \leq V2\%$. The average volumes amounted to CTV-T = 198 ± 120 cm^3, PTV-T = 475 ± 180 cm^3, CTV-N = 334 ± 140 cm^3, and PTV-TN = 1323 ± 300 cm^3.

The first-stage EBRT dosimetric treatment planning was carried out in the XIO dosimetry planning system (version 5.1, Elekta AB) using the conventional RT ^{60}Co with Theratron Equinox 100 gamma apparatus and 3D-CRT technique at the Elekta Synergy linac at 10 MeV. Dosimetric planning of conventional RT ^{60}Co and 3D-CRT was carried out using the superposition calculation algorithm based on modified four-field irradiation. For conventional RT, lateral irradiation on the right and left was complemented by the "field-in-field" irradiation technique and the distribution of weight dose loads to improve the target coverage. For 3D-CRT, the upper and lower fields were divided into subfields with turns at gantry angles of 340° and 20° to reduce the radiation load on the OARs while keeping an acceptable level of target coverage.

The first-stage EBRT dosimetric treatment planning based on the VMAT technique was carried out using the Monaco dosimetric planning system (v. 5.10.04, Elekta) at the Elekta Synergy linac at 10 MeV. For the VMAT technique, the inverse algorithms based on the Monte Carlo method were used. The dose delivery was realized using three full arches. The grid step was 0.3 cm, the minimum width of the segment was 1 cm, and the uncertainty of the entire calculation was 0.8% during the dose simulation.

In **Table 2**, one can see the results of dosimetric planning of the first-stage EBRT averaged over all patients.

Dose, %	^{60}Co, V%	3D-CRT, V%	VMAT, V%
90	97.9 [96.9–99.0]	99.2 [99.0–99.4]	98.8 [98.4–99.2]
95	89.0 [85.6–92.3]	95.7 [95.2–96.2]	97.0 [96.1–97.9]
98	72.7 [64.0–81.4]	87.2 [85.3–89.0]	93.5 [91.5–95.5]
99	62.1 [50.8–73.4]	81.5 [78.5–84.4]	90.4 [87.0–93.7]
100	47.9 [34.8–60.9]	71.8 [66.5–77.1]	84.5 [78.9–90.1]
110	0 [0–0]	0 [0–0]	1.5 [0–4.4]

Table 2.
PTV-TN dose coverage for the first stage of combined RT.

From **Table 2**, one can see that, as expected, the use of a more complex and higher gradient dose delivery technique (VMAT) leads to an increase in the irradiation of the tumor and the regional-iliac lymph nodes. The VMAT method allows reaching the level of coverage of 95% of the prescribed dose delivered in 97% of the irradiation volume, which can be considered a very good indicator of the coverage uniformity. It should be noted, however, that even the use of a conventional RT ^{60}Co on a gamma device allows one to confidently exceed the coverage level of 90% of the prescribed dose delivered to 90% of the irradiation volume, ensuring even the level of 90% of the dose to 97.9% of the volume. At the same time, for 95% of the prescribed dose, the average irradiated volume is 89%, which should also be recognized as a good result for the conventional ^{60}Co technique. The 3D-CRT technique allows obtaining a coverage level of 95–95%, which fully satisfies the prescription.

2.2 HDR for the second stage

To prepare for HDR BT, the patients were scanned using the CT scanner in a supine position with inserted Manchester-type CT-compatible implants (rigid direct central intrauterine endostat and two rigid lateral intrauterine endostats with ovoid) that were sufficiently fixed.

CT scans give poor visualization of the tumor, which is why the whole uterus (whole cervix) was chosen as CTV for BT (CTV-B). No additional safety margins are needed to take into account internal movement during BT because the applicator moves together with the CTV [2–5]. Although there are some uncertainties for setup (applicator reconstruction), these seem to be rather negligible, if the systematic error can be kept below 2 mm and the slice thickness below 5 mm (random error) [3]. In the present study, we assumed that no margins should be added to CTV-B, resulting in CTV-B = PTV-B.

For compensation of possible changes of target and OAR localization with respect to the position of the applicator, each BT implant insertion was followed by a new CT study with the applicator in situ and a new dose plan calculation. Contouring for both CTV and OARs was performed for each insertion/implant of BT applicators.

The treatment planning goal for HDR BT was prescribed to deliver more than 90% of the dose to 90% of the volume (D90% ≥ V90%). DVHs were used for the analysis of the planning results.

The dose limitations to OARs were set for the bladder and rectum according to the limits listed in **Table 1**. The whole organs were contoured based on CT images without division on parts.

For OAR, it was important to specify the position of the hot spots in the bladder (D_{2cc}) because this small volume may have an impact on the clinical outcome, and so delineation of full organs based on CT images and dose was estimated in any location whose accordance did not exceed the tolerance level (see **Table 1**).

The dosimetric planning of the HDR BT of the second stage was carried out using the HDRplus 3D BT dose-planning system (version 3.4) for the MultiSource HDR apparatus with ^{60}Co source (Bebig, Germany).

During the planning procedure, the implant was carefully reconstructed, and the conventional standard loading pattern matching the prescribed dose to point A was applied. From this starting point, dose optimization was performed with the goal of adapting the dose to the CTV-B. The optimization of CTV-B dose coverage and OAR dose constraints was carried out using the following steps:

- Dose point optimization
- Manual dwell time or dwell weight optimization
- Graphical optimization ("dose shaping") combined with manual verification and adjustments for unnecessarily large deviations from standard loading patterns

There is the task of summation of the doses from the first-stage EBRT and the second-stage HDR BT. This was done based on the assumptions given by GYN GEC ESTRO recommendation [3]. According to Ref. [3], it is assumed that CTV and OARs receive the full dose from the EBRT course. Thus, it was assumed that the dose in the small volumes of interest for BT (anterior-lateral walls of the rectum and sigmoid, posterior-inferior wall of the bladder, and wall of the vagina adjacent to macroscopic disease) receives the EBRT prescribed dose for CTV-T and CTV-N.

2.3 VMAT for the second stage

The VMAT technique with three full arches was used as EBRT of the second stage. The dosimetric planning was carried out using the same CT scans as for the first-stage EBRT because no specific patient scanning was done after the first-stage EBRT. The PTV tumor for the second stage was assumed to be equal to CTV-T of the first stage plus 5 mm safety margin. In our opinion, it is sufficient estimation, taking into account the fact that the tumor shrinks after the first-stage EBRT.

The second-stage VMAT dosimetric planning was carried out using the Monaco dosimetric planning system (v. 5.10.04, Elekta) at the Elekta Synergy linac at 10 MeV. For the VMAT technique, the inverse algorithms based on the Monte Carlo method were used. The dose delivery was realized using three full arches. The grid step was 0.3 cm, the minimum width of the segment was 1 cm, and the uncertainty of the entire calculation was 0.8% during the dose simulation.

2.4 Summation of the first- and second-stage results

When planning a combined RT in the EBRT + BT format, the question of DVH summation arises because the DVHs were calculated by different planning systems that are completely incompatible. Therefore, we assumed that during the first stage, the CTV-T was irradiated uniformly up to the prescribed dose of 50 Gy. The DVH from the second-stage HDR BT was added to that dose value [2–6]. The damage to the OARs was assessed by the criterion of the total EQD_2 delivered to 2 cm^3 from both courses of EBRT and HDR BT because the summation of DVHs for OARs is illegal because of OAR shape changes while inserting the implants [2–5, 18]. For combined therapy in the EBRT + VMAT format, the EQD_2 DVHs from the EBRT and VMAT course were summed up for CTV-T and OARs.

3. Results and discussion

Figure 1 shows examples of the planned dose distribution for the first and second stages of combined radiotherapy.

Let us further consider the results of the total combined RT course. **Figure 1** shows an example of DVHs for CTV-T, for one of the patients. **Figure 2** shows all considered irradiation combinations (3D-CRT + HDR-BT, ^{60}Co + VMAT, 3D-CRT + VMAT, VMAT + VMAT).

In **Figure 2**, one can see that with the use of HDR BT, the dose distribution over the target volume is nonuniform, i.e., there are proportions of the volume of radiation that receive doses substantially higher than prescribed.

Table 3 shows the resulting dose coverage for the total treatment course as the mean value obtained for 11 patients and a confidence interval [27].

From **Table 3**, one can see that combined RT based on HDR BT results in 90% of prescribed dose delivered to 95.9% of the target volume, which is a rather good result. However, HDR BT results in irradiation of the significant target volumes by doses that are significantly higher than the prescribed dose. In this case, 150–200% of the prescribed dose was delivered to 44.6 and 19.7% of the volume, respectively.

The use of VMAT as the second stage of the combined RT significantly improves the situation. Regardless of the dose delivery technique used during the first stage dose, 95% of the prescribed dose is delivered to 97% of the volume. The hot spots do not exceed 110% of the prescribed dose delivered in less than 9% of the volume for the VMAT + VMAT combination. It should be noted that even the use of the conventional RT based on ^{60}Co in combination with VMAT allows one to achieve such a high level of target coverage.

Figure 3 shows examples of bladder and rectum DVHs in the case of the VMAT technique used as the second stage of combined RT. Statistical data on the irradiation of critical organs are given in **Table 4** for the bladder and in **Table 5** for the rectum.

From **Table 4**, one can see that the dose load on the bladder using ^{60}Co + VMAT or VMAT + VMAT combinations allows meeting the tolerant levels, avoiding third-degree radiation complications (see **Table 1**). For the combination of 3D-CRT + VMAT, there is a slight exceeding of the tolerant levels for the dose levels of 65 Gy and 70 Gy. This dose overload is caused by the high level of the dose coverage during the first stage when 95% of the prescribed dose was delivered to 95% of the volume (see **Table 2**). In the case of conventional irradiation, the dose load meets the tolerant levels because the first-stage dose coverage is lower than the 95–95% prescription. The use of VMAT techniques reduces the dose loads due to modulation of the radiation intensity.

According to the criterion of the maximum dose delivered to the volume of 2 cm^3 of the bladder, all the methods of dose delivery meet the constraints, although the best result was obtained with the use of HDR BT. When using VMAT + VMAT technology, there are individual cases exceeding the tolerant dose of 90 Gy per 2 cm^3 volume, which is caused by escalation of the dose in the target. In this case, it is difficult to judge whether this will lead to radiation complications because the irradiation levels of parts of the bladder do not exceed the tolerant levels of QUANTEC.

Table 5 shows the radiation loads on the rectum for the different combinations of dose delivery techniques. From **Table 5**, one can see that the use of the VMAT + VMAT combination does not exceed the tolerance levels established by the

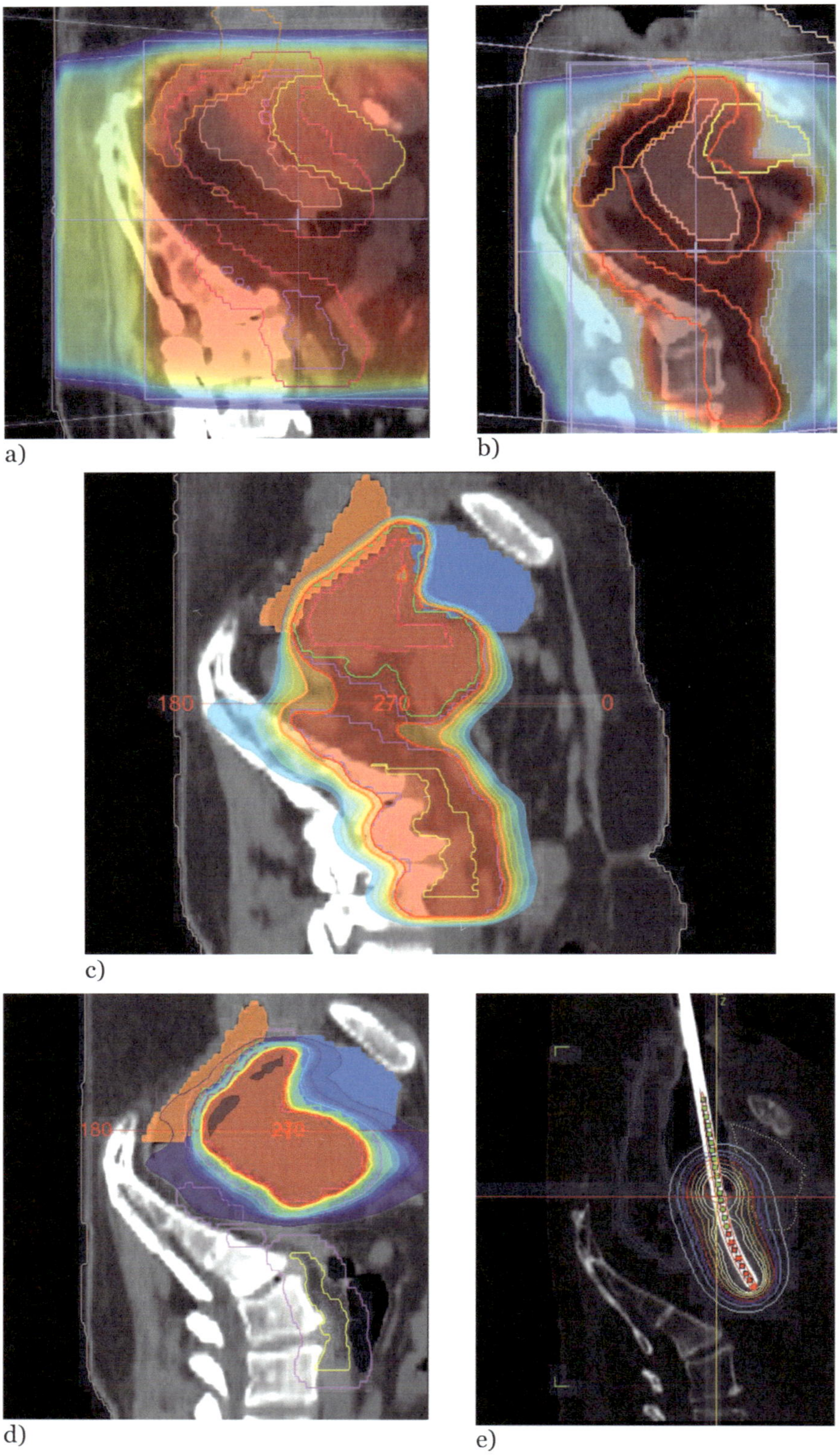

Figure 1.
Dose distributions of treatment plans: (a) ^{60}Co, (b) 3D-CRT, (c) VMAT for the first stage, (d) VMAT for the second stage, and (e) HDR.

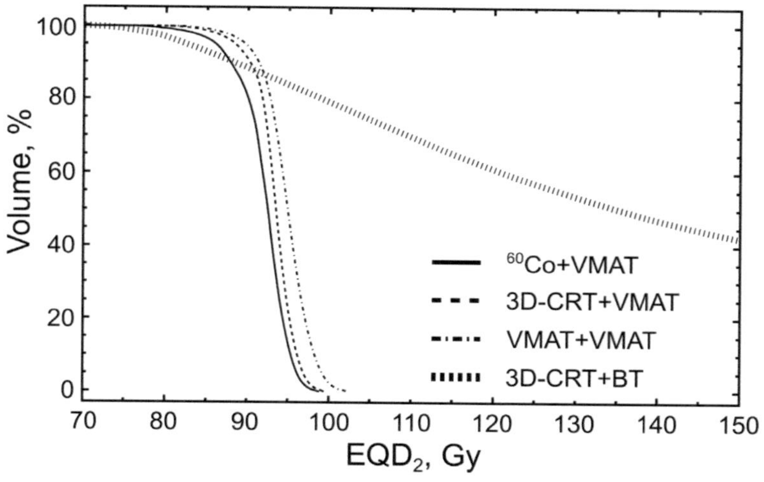

Figure 2.
Example of DVHs calculated for target volume for different variants of combined therapy at prescribed dose EQD2 = 89.7 Gy.

Dose, %	3D-CRT + BT, volume %	^{60}Co + VMAT, v %	3D-CRT + VMAT, volume %	VMAT+VMAT, volume %
90	95.9 [94.8–96.9]	99.3 [98.9–99.6]	99.6 [99.4–99.8]	99.7 [99.6–99.8]
95	91.8 [90.5–93.2]	97.1 [96.1–98.0]	98.0 [97.4–98.5]	98.8 [98.4–99.3]
98	88.8 [87.2–90.3]	92.4 [90.4–94.3]	94.7 [93.3–96.0]	97.0 [96.1–97.9]
99	87.7 [86.1–89.4]	89.4 [86.8–91.9]	92.5 [90.6–94.4]	95.8 [94.6–97.0]
100	86.7 [85.0–88.4]	85.0 [81.4–88.7]	89.2 [86.6–91.8]	93.9 [92.2–95.5]
110	75.7 [73.3–78.2]	2.1 [0.9–3.4]	2.6 [1.2–4.1]	8.8 [5.4–12.1]
150	44.6 [41.8–47.4]	—	—	—
200	27.4 [25.2–29.6]	—	—	—
250	19.7 [17.7–21.6]	—	—	—

Table 3.
Target coverage for different courses of combined RT.

QUANTEC protocol. In the case of ^{60}Co + VMAT and 3D-CRT + VMAT combinations, there is an exceeding of tolerant levels. In these cases, 60 Gy EQD_2 is delivered to more than 35% of the volume and 50 Gy EQD_2 to more than 50%. This can lead to late second- and third-grade complications. Such results appear due to large irradiation volumes. During the first-stage irradiation, PTV is close to the anterior rectal wall, which leads to its irradiation. The use of the VMAT technique allows reducing the radiation load during the implementation of high-gradient plans. To reduce the exposure of the rectum, it is necessary to reduce the margin between

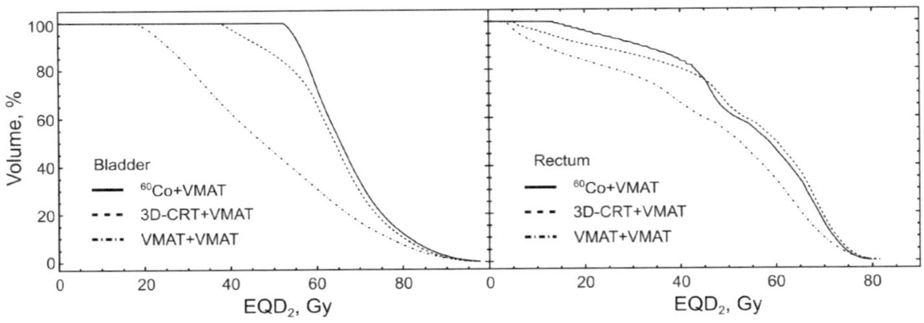

Figure 3.
Example of DVHs calculated for bladder and rectum for one of the patients.

EQD$_2$/volume % QUANTEC	3D-CRT + BT, volume %	^{60}Co + VMAT, volume %	3D-CRT + VMAT, volume %	VMAT+VMAT, volume %
80 Gy/15%	—	12.1 [7.1–17.0]	12.7 [7.4–18.0]	11.8 [7.0–16.6]
75 Gy/25%	—	19.7 [13.6–25.9]	23.3 [15.3–31.4]	18.6 [12.5–24.7]
70 Gy/35%	—	29.1 [22.1–36.1]	37.0 [26.5–47.5]	26.0 [19.1–32.8]
65 Gy/50%	—	40.4 [31.4–49.5]	52.3 [41.4–63.2]	33.5 [26.2–40.8]
Volume	3D-CRT + BT, EQD$_2$, Gy	^{60}Co + VMAT, EQD$_2$, Gy	3D-CRT + VMAT, EQD$_2$, Gy	VMAT+VMAT, EQD$_2$, Gy
2 cm^3 < 90 Gy EQD$_2$	82.2 [74.6–89.8]	87.2 [84.4–90.0]	87.7 [85.0–90.4]	88.9 [85.8–92.2]

Table 4.
Bladder dose loads for different courses of combined RT.

EQD$_2$/volume % QUANTEC	3D-CRT + BT, volume %	^{60}Co + VMAT, volume %	3D-CRT + VMAT, volume %	VMAT+VMAT, volume %
75 Gy/15%	—	2.6 [0.9–4.3]	2.5 [0.9–4.0]	2.1 [1.2–3.0]
70 Gy/20%	—	9.4 [3.9–15.0]	8.5 [3.3–13.7]	6 [3.4–8.6]
65 Gy/25%	—	22.3 [12.4–33.3]	20.3 [9.8–30.7]	13.2 [7.8–18.5]
60 Gy/ 35%	—	42.1 [30.1–54.2]	38.4 [25.5–51.3]	22.6 [15.4–29.9]
50 Gy/ 50%	—	77.3 [67.9–86.8]	73.3 [65.0–81.7]	44.3 [35.4–53.1]
Volume	3D-CRT + BT, EQD$_2$, Gy	^{60}Co + VMAT, EQD$_2$, Gy	3D-CRT + VMAT, EQD$_2$, Gy	VMAT+VMAT, EQD$_2$, Gy
2 cm^3 < 75 Гр EQD$_2$	70.9 [67.1–74.7]	71.9 [69.5–74.4]	72.4 [69.9–74.9]	71.5 [69.3–73.7]

Table 5.
Rectum dose loads for different courses of combined RT.

PTV-T and CTV-T for the displacement of organs, which requires fixing the position of the target, the rectum, and the stability of the filling of the bladder.

In **Table 5**, one can see that there is no exceeding of the rectum tolerant level by 2 cm^3 parameter for any combination of the techniques simulated. It should again be noted that the criterion of 2 cm^3 has a much lower accuracy than the DVH estimate.

The combined RT for cervical cancer can be realized using different combinations of the first- and second-stage irradiation techniques. The efficiency of the total course can be analyzed using two parameters, which are dose coverage of the target (both tumor and nodes during the first stage) and the dose loads on the OARs.

Thus, from the point of view of target coverage, the ^{60}Co + VMAT and 3D-CRT + VMAT combinations are very similar because with ^{60}Co + VMAT, coverage is 95% of the prescribed dose, 97.1% of the volume, and with 3D-CRT + VMAT, 95% of the dose, 98% of the volume. Unfortunately, the use of the gamma apparatus loses in the first stage of the combined RT because the coverage of the volume of PTV is only 95% of the dose—89% of the volume—and with 3D-CRT 95% of the dose, 95.1% of the volume. Despite this, it can be pointed out that using a gamma apparatus for EBRT can be effective for a combined RT when followed by VMAT, providing good coverage of the target with a 10–15% chance of late second- and third-grade complications to the rectum and bladder. When using the VMAT + VMAT combination, a coverage level of 98–97% is achieved without exceeding the tolerant levels for all critical organs.

Obviously, the values of radiation loads will depend on the accuracy of contour creation for both the target and for critical organs, as well as the offset space used. Therefore, the results of irradiation substantially depend on the degree of immobilization of the patient, which includes maintaining the mutual position of the internal organs by introducing a Foley catheter, as well as minimizing and controlling their displacement during breathing (e.g., abdominal press).

The main advantage of using the VMAT technique for the second stage of combined RT is to simplify the treatment procedure, to reduce the painful sensations typical for BT in the process of topometric preparation and treatment, as well as to reduce the time of the irradiation session. When using VMAT technology, the radiotherapist's labor costs (no need for implants) are reduced, but the work of the topometrist (the need for more accurate contouring) and the medical physicist (more complex dosimetric planning and the need for dosimetry quality assurance) increases.

One of the effective ways to implement the use of the VMAT technique for the second-stage irradiation is to use both CT and MRI for the topographic preparation of the patient after the first-stage irradiation.

4. Conclusion

In the considered examples, it can be seen that the use of the VMAT dose delivery technique for the second stage of combined RT of cervical cancer allows a significant increase in the irradiation uniformity, to exclude overexposure of large volumes with high doses (more than 115% of the prescribed dose) and to deliver the prescribed dose to the target with a high coverage level (95.8% of the target volume can be irradiated with a dose higher than 99% of the prescribed dose), not exceeding the dose loads to OARs.

In Tomsk Regional Oncology Center, HDR brachytherapy is not fully equipped by implants of different types needed for effective treatment of the cervical cancer. Also we do not have the equipment for the gynecological interstitial brachytherapy that significantly limits our possibilities. At the same time, Tomsk Regional Oncology Center has good competences in the EBRT VMAT treatment planning, QA, and delivery. The results of presented study show that the VMAT dose delivery could be effective enough to replace HDR brachytherapy in some case.

There are different patients that could benefit from the change of HDR BT to VMAT. These are the patients with challenging cervical dilation, perforation risk, patients with asymmetric tumor invasion, and patients with personal reasons to avoid the BT procedure.

The results of this study that have shown the technical possibility of HDR BT replacement were the basis to start this method in the clinical practice. These days, five patients are treated with VMAT for the second stage of combined radiotherapy with cisplatin chemotherapy. The patients chosen have intolerance to procedure, asymmetric tumor invasion, and religious contradictions to the intracavitary BT.

Due to the focus of the present study on the dosimetric and radiobiological evaluation of the radiotherapy using different dose delivery techniques, we cannot discuss the advantages of the different treatment methods that include surgery, adjuvant or neoadjuvant therapy, etc. These treatment modalities should be carefully examined for each patient. In the case when RT can be performed, the HDR BT could be examined to the possibility to be replaced by the VMAT technique. In this case, it does not matter which treatment modality is used, postsurgery + EBRT, chemotherapy + EBRT, etc.

Author details

Evgeniia Sergeevna Sukhikh[1,2]* and Leonid Grigorievich Sukhikh[2]

1 Medical Physics Department, Tomsk Regional Oncology Centre, Tomsk, Russia

2 Research School of Physics of High-Energy Processes, Tomsk Polytechnic University, Tomsk, Russia

*Address all correspondence to: e.s.sukhikh@gmail.com

References

[1] Kravchenko GR, Zharov AV, Vazhenin AV, et al. Results of multicomponent treatment of patients with locally advanced forms of cervical cancer. Siberian Oncological Journal. 2009;**33**(3):20-23. Russian

[2] Kravets OA, Andreeva YV, Kozlov OV, Nechushkin MI. Clinical and radiobiological planning of brachytherapy of locally advanced cervical cancer. Medical Physics. 2009; **33**(2):10-17. Russian

[3] A European Study on MRI-Guided Brachytherapy in Locally Advanced Cervical Cancer EMBRACE. 2009. Available from: https://www.embracestudy.dk/UserUpload/PublicDocuments/EmbraceProtocol.pdf [Accessed: 22 July 2019]

[4] Hellebust TA, Kirisits C, Berger D. Recommendations for gynaecological (GYN) GEC ESTRO working group: Considerations and pitfalls in commissioning and applicator reconstruction in 3D image-based treatment planning of cervix cancer brachytherapy. Radiotherapy and Oncology. 2010;**96**(2):153-160. DOI: 10.1016/j.radonc.2010.06.004

[5] Kravets OA, Kozlov OV, Fedyanina AA, et al. Methodical aspects of contact radiation therapy of cervical cancer using 3D-planning. Medical Physics. 2017;**73**(1):16-24. Russian

[6] Banerjee R, Kamrava M. Brachytherapy in the treatment of cervical cancer: A review. International Journal of Women's Health. 2014;**6**:555-564

[7] Vishwanathan AN, Beriwal S, De Los Santos JF. American brachytherapy society consensus guidelines for locally advanced carcinoma of the cervix. Part II: High-dose-rate brachytherapy. Brachytherapy. 2012;**11**(1):47-52. DOI: 10.1016/j.brachy.2011.07.002

[8] Bucci MK, Bevan A, Roach M. Advances in radiation therapy: Conventional to 3D, to IMRT, to 4D and beyond. CA: A Cancer Journal for Clinicians. 2005;**55**(2):117-134. PubMed PMID: 15761080

[9] Roeske JC, Lujan A, Rotmensch J, Waggoner SE, Yamada D, Mundt AJ. Intensity-modulated whole pelvic radiation therapy in patients with gynecologic malignancies. International Journal of Radiation Oncology, Biology, Physics. 2000;**48**(5):1613-1621

[10] Chernyaev AP, Popodko AI, Lykova EN. Medical Equipment in the Modern Radiotherapy. Moscow, Russian: MSU Physical Faculty Publishing; 2019. 101 p

[11] Roitberg GE, Usychkin SV, Boyko AV. Large-scale remote radiation therapy for prostate cancer. Medical Radiology and Radiation Safety. 2016; **61**(1):47-59. Russian

[12] Ghandour S, Matzinger O, Pachouda M. Volumetric-modulated arc therapy planning using multicriteria optimization for localized prostate cancer. Journal of Applied Clinical Medical Physics. 2015;**16**(3):258-269. DOI: 10.1120/jacmp.v16i3.5410

[13] Rodríguez Villalba S, Planell CD, Grau JM. Current opinion in cervix carcinoma. Clinical and Translational Oncology. 2011;**13**:378-384. DOI: 10.1007/s12094-011-0671-4

[14] Chan P, Yeo I, Perkins G, Fyles A, Milosevic M. Dosimetric comparison of intensity-modulated, conformal, and four-field pelvic radiotherapy boost plans for gynecologic cancer: A retrospective planning study. Radiation Oncology. 2006;**1**:13. DOI: 10.1186/1748-717X-1-13

[15] Cozzia L, Dinshawc KA, Shrivastavac SK, Mahantshettyc U,

Engineerc R, Deshpandec DD, et al. A treatment planning study comparing volumetric arc modulation with RapidArc and fixed field IMRT for cervix uteri radiotherapy. Radiotherapy and Oncology. 2008;**89**:180-191

[16] Khosla D, Patel FD, Oinam AS, Tomar P, Sharma SC. Dosimetric comparison of vaginal vault ovoid brachytherapy versus intensity-modulated radiation therapy plans in postoperative patients of cervical carcinoma following whole pelvic radiotherapy. Journal of Cancer Research and Therapeutics. 2014;**10**(1): 153-158. DOI: 10.4103/0973-1482.131449

[17] Pedicini P, Caivano R, Fiorentino A, Strigari L, Califano G, Barbieri V, et al. Comparative dosimetric and radiobiological assessment among a nonstandard RapidArc, standard RapidArc, classical intensity-modulated radiotherapy, and 3D brachytherapy for the treatment of the vaginal vault in patients affected by gynecologic cancer. Medical Dosimetry. 2012;**37**(4):347-352. DOI: 10.1016/j.meddos.2011.11.009

[18] Mahmoud O, Kilic S, Khan AJ, Beriwal S, Small W Jr. External beam techniques to boost cervical cancer when brachytherapy is not an option—Theories and applications. The Annals of Translational Medicine. 2017;**5**(10): 207. DOI: 10.21037/atm.2017.03.102

[19] Cihoric N, Tsikkinis A, Miguelez CG, Strnad V, Soldatovic I, Ghadjar P, et al. Portfolio of prospective clinical trials including brachytherapy: An analysis of the ClinicalTrials.gov database. Radiation Oncology. 2016; **22**(11):48. DOI: 10.1186/s13014-016-0624-8.

[20] Mell LK, Mundt AJ. Intensity-modulated radiation therapy in gynecologic cancers: Growing support, growing acceptance. Cancer Journal. 2008;**14**(3):198-199. DOI: 10.1097/PPO.0b013e318178dda1

[21] Cilla S, Macchia G, Sabatino D, Digesù C, Deodato F, Piermattei A, De Spirito M, Morganti AG. Applicator-guided volumetric-modulated arc therapy for low-risk endometrial cancer. Medical Dosimetry 2013;38(1):5–11. DOI: 10.1016/j.meddos.2012.04.004

[22] Assenholt MS, Petersen JB, Nielsen SK, Lindegaard JC, Tanderup K. A dose planning study on applicator guided stereotactic IMRT boost in combination with 3D MRI based brachytherapy in locally advanced cervical cancer. Acta Oncologica. 2008; **47**(7):1337. DOI: 10.1080/02841860802266698

[23] Michalski JM, Gay H, Jackson A, Tucker SL, Deasy JO. Radiation dose-volume effects in radiation-induced rectal injury. International Journal of Radiation Oncology, Biology, Physics. 2010;**76**(3):123. DOI: 10.1016/j.ijrobp.2009.03.078

[24] Viswanathan AN, Yorke ED, Marks LB, Eifel PJ, Shipley WU. Radiation dose–volume effects of the urinary bladder. International Journal of Radiation Oncology, Biology, Physics. 2010;**76**(3):116-S122. DOI: 10.1016/j.ijrobp.2009.02.090

[25] RTOG/EORTC Late Radiation Morbidity Scoring Schema. Available from: https://www.rtog.org/ResearchAssociates/AdverseEventReporting/RTOGEORTCLateRadiationMorbidityScoringSchema.aspx [Accessed: 22 July 2019]

[26] Georg P, Pötter R, Georg D, Lang S, Dimopoulos JC, Sturdza AE, et al. Dose effect relationship for late side effects of the rectum and urinary bladder in magnetic resonance image-guided adaptive cervix cancer brachytherapy. International Journal of Radiation

Oncology, Biology, Physics. 2012;**82**(2): 653. DOI: 10.1016/j.ijrobp.2010.12.029

[27] Gmurman VE. Theory of Probability and Mathematical Statistics. 9th ed. Moscow: Higher School; 2003. 479 p. Russian

Chapter 6

Intraoperative Radiation Therapy in Gynecological Cancer

Albert Biete, Angeles Rovirosa and Gabriela Oses

Abstract

Gynecological malignancies, mainly cervical uterine cancer, continue to present a high number of pelvic and para-aortic recurrences. Intraoperative radiation therapy (IORT) allows a precise therapeutic boost in the surgical bed in the cases in which removal of the tumor relapse is feasible. At the same time, IORT permits the exclusion of the radiosensitive organs from the irradiation field. While the first published gynecological IORT took place in 1905, the number of patients per year became stable and the published series are retrospective and limited. Recurrences are located in different areas with non-homogeneous prognostic and most of the published manuscripts are retrospective including a mix of primaries, sites and different types and results of salvage surgery. We have revised the present knowledge in this field and the main conclusion is that IORT increases the local control and, in selected cases, probably slightly the survival. Also, the quality of life is probably increased. Randomized trials that allow a breakthrough in the conclusions are highly unlikely to be performed in recurrent gynecological malignancies.

Keywords: gynecological cancer, radiotherapy, intraoperative radiation therapy, uterine cancer, ovarian cancer, endometrial cancer

1. Background

Intraoperative radiation therapy (IORT) is a boosting technique that delivers a single high dose fraction of radiation directly to the resection bed during surgery. The purpose is to selectively irradiate anatomical areas that have been identified as high risk of persistence of subclinical disease or even macroscopic unresectable residual disease. This identification is easily achieved by the direct vision of the area of interest through the surgical field. At the same time, IORT protects or avoids damage to surrounding structures or organs at risk (OAR) because they are radiosensitive. This allows good protection of pelvic organs, such as urinary bladder, ureter, rectum, bowel, etc., and, consequently, decreases the incidence of secondary undesired effects including enteritis, proctitis or cystitis. IORT can be delivered using a dedicated linear accelerator producing electron beams of different energies and penetration degrees, X-ray sources delivering low-energy radiation or high dose-rate brachytherapy sources. All of them can also be conveniently used for IORT procedures in primary or recurrent gynecological tumors. All techniques have different advantages and disadvantages. In the initial period, conventional radiotherapy linear accelerators were used, which meant that the patient had to be moved from the operating room to the radiotherapy room, which was sometimes far away. Apart from inconveniences to transfer the patient at the time of surgery, there was also a risk of infections and a substantial prolongation of surgery time. As a result, compact mobile electron accelerators were designed that could be installed in a radio-protected operating room to avoid patient transfer (Mobetron and LIAC are the best known). Low kilovoltage X-ray tubes, such as Intrabeam, have a more specific design for intraoperative breast radiotherapy and do not have collimators of sufficient diameter. Another added difficulty is that the irradiation time is too long, about 20–40 minutes as compared to a few minutes in electron accelerators. Also, several dosimetric considerations are favoring the use of accelerated electron beams over 50 kV X-ray beams, the description of which is out of the scope of this chapter.

In the Radiation Oncology literature, the first description of an IORT procedure has been consistently attributed to Beck [1] but Casals et al. [2] from Barcelona documented a case of an IORT treatment in the gynecological area some years before. Comas and Prio [3] reported the case of a 33-year-old woman diagnosed with a cervical squamous cell carcinoma treated by radical surgery and intrapelvic roentgen therapy to the left parametria. The patient survived at least 6 years after the treatment was completed (**Figure 1**). Results were very limited for much of the century, but through the introduction of megavoltage linear accelerators and later specifically designed units as previously explained, studies of IORT delivery procedures began to be published.

IORT has been used in the primary management, as well as in the salvage setting, for many solid tumors of different locations. Conservative treatment of breast cancer has been the most common indication, but many treatments have been done in other sites such as the pancreas, the rectum, the cardio-esophageal junction, etc.

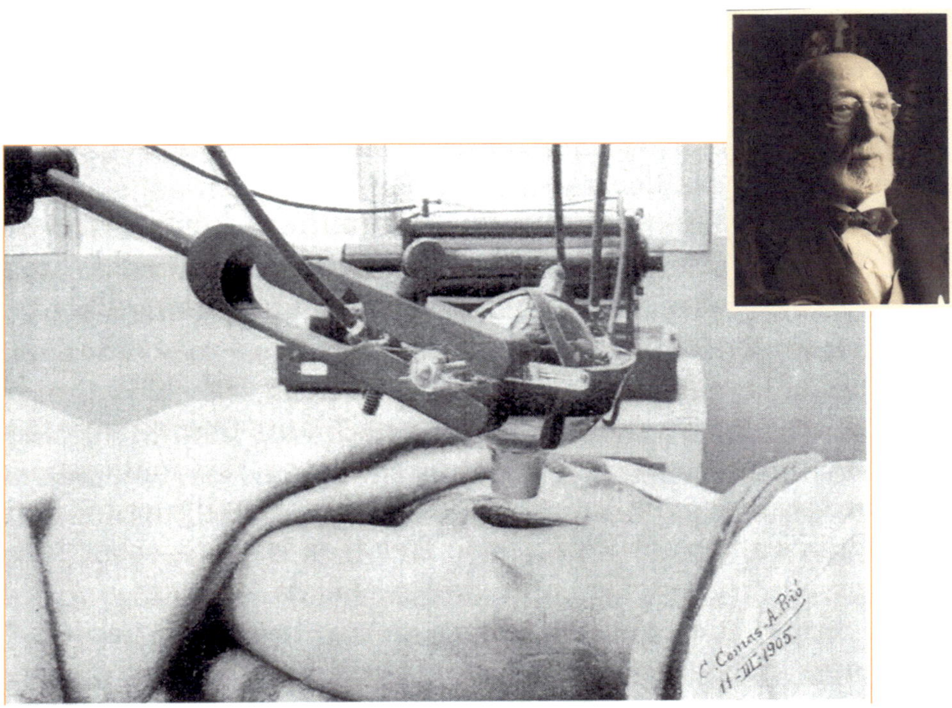

Figure 1.
Original picture of the first published IORT treatment. The patient was irradiated to the distant parametrial area and survived at least 7 years. Drs. C. comas and A. Prio signed the image. Barcelona, 1905.

Two reviews on IORT in gynecological tumors have been previously published. The first one, from Backes and Martin [4], comprises all gynecological malignancies, including separate sections focused on uterine primary tumors and recurrent cervical cancer. A total amount of 276 cases of cervical cancer (primary and recurrent) were collected. The main conclusion is that if the surgical margins are positive or close, IORT appears to increase local control of the disease, with an acceptable toxicity profile. The second review, recently published by Krengly et al. [5], focuses on endometrial, cervical, renal, bladder and prostate cancers. A total of 153 patients (primary and recurrent cervical cancer) from 4 studies are analyzed in detail. They conclude as follows: in recurrent cervical cancer from these studies, it emerged that the status of the margins is the most important risk factor for treatment and the association of IORT seems to improve the probability of local control. In contrast, they do not recommend surgery and IORT for primary tumors. They state: "The available data suggests that this aggressive strategy is not advantageous in particular for the risk of severe side effects and that concomitant radio-chemotherapy alone should be considered the best treatment strategy in this patient setting."

2. Biological and technical considerations

IORT using a linear accelerator of mobile electrons is given by applying a set of collimators of different diameters to the area of interest. The distal end may be perpendicular to the longitudinal or oblique axis, facilitating access to areas in the pelvic wall. The rotation of the accelerator head makes it easier to adapt the collimator to the area to be irradiated. If a risk organ cannot move out of the irradiation field, it can be protected by a metal disc, which is interposed between it and the radiation beam. The available accelerated electron energies are in a range of 4–12 MeV and the available collimator diameters are between 4 and 8 cm. The electron beams deposit their energy to a depth between 1.5 and 4 cm depending on the energy used. The dose refers to the 90% isodoses and from the determined depth falls sharply, which protects the organs located deeper. IORT can also be given employing Ir-192 thread brachytherapy, but it is a more complex procedure and requires more time, and radioprotection, as well as the surface dose/dose ratio at the desired depth, is more unfavorable (**Figure 2**).

The carcinogenic effect depends not only on the nature of the radiation but also on the total dose and the time in which it is given (relative biological efficacy, RBE). The conventional dose per session in external pelvic radiotherapy is 1.8–2 Grays (Gy). In IORT, the doses usually used are 10–20 Gy and it is estimated that the RBE of this single large dose is equivalent up to 2–3 times the dose if delivered as standard external beam radiotherapy. Consequently, IORT can deliver more effective radiotherapy than an external beam, because the antineoplastic efficacy is strongly related to the dose.

Also, there is probably an extra benefit coming from diminishing the release of cell growth-stimulating cytokines. This has been well reported by Belletti et al. [6] in 2008 and later by Zaleska et al. [7] in 2016. It was shown that the growth of cell cultures of breast cancer lines could be stimulated by adding the fluid collected from the operative field to cell cultures. By contrast, if the fluid was collected after irradiation of the surgical site, no such stimulus was elicited. This may help to explain the high effectiveness of IORT in preventing tumor recurrence in the treated area. Also, it has been shown that irradiation blocks the proliferative cascade induced by surgical wound repair. Moreover, Zaleska et al. [7] showed that inhibition patterns vary according to the different histological types of breast cancer, with maximum inhibition in the luminal subtypes.

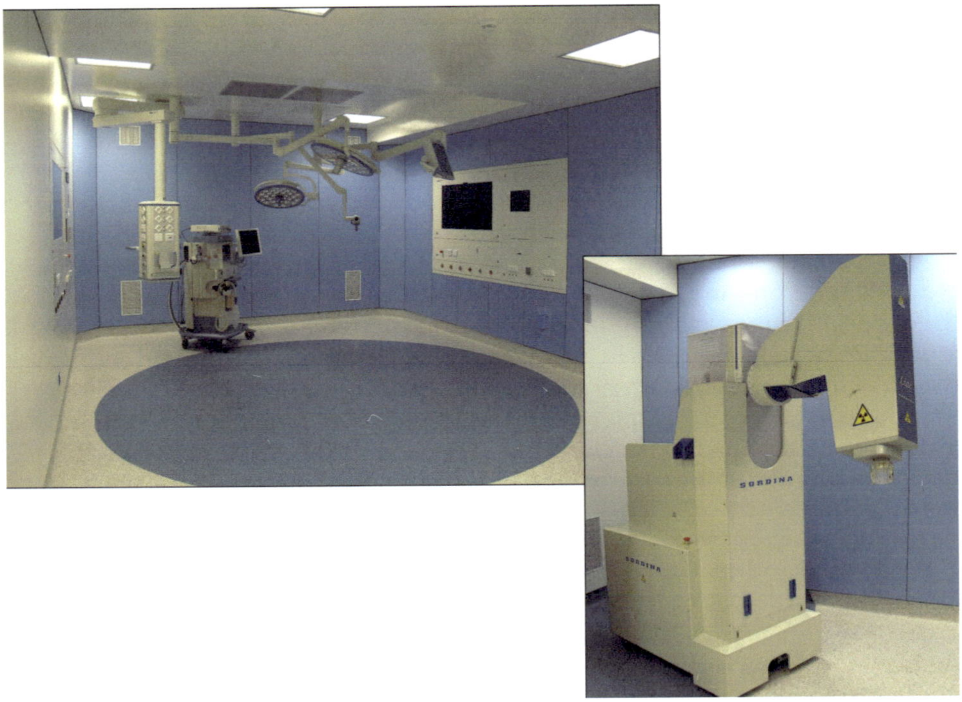

Figure 2.
Operating room designed for IORT and equipped with a mobile electron linear accelerator (LIAC). Hospital clinic. The University of Barcelona.

3. Intraoperative radiotherapy in locally advanced cervical cancer

The elective treatment in advanced cervical cancer is simultaneous radiochemotherapy followed by brachytherapy plus/minus parametrial depending on the extend of the tumor after chemoradiation. Nevertheless, in some cases, brachytherapy could not be performed and then these patients could be treated using SBRT (Stereotaxic radiotherapy) techniques but with lower results in comparison to the elective treatment. Although in 2/3 of the patients the clinical results are satisfactory, there are some cases in which the tumor remains out of control. IORT has been considered a novel approach after the removal of the persistent tumor to boost with irradiation of the surgical bed at risk and mainly performed in FIGO stages IIB.

Martinez-Monge et al. [8] described in 31 patients the results of IORT after surgery in resectable cervical cancer. These patients were treated from 1986 to 1999 with cisplatin plus fluorouracil chemotherapy simultaneously with pelvic irradiation (dose: 45 Gy). After tumor removal, IORT was delivered to the risk areas [mainly pelvic sidewalls with a median dose of 12 Gy (range between 10 and 25 Gy)]. Patients were irradiated using electrons of 9 or 12 MeV and the median field size was 6.4 cm (range between 5 and 12 cm). The 10-year local control obtained in the irradiation field was 92.8% and the pelvic control 78.6%. Attributable to IORT, toxicity was found in 14% of the patients manifested as transient pelvic pain and only one patient had neuropathy. The authors considered IORT as a boosting technique feasible and valuable in advanced resectable cervical tumors.

Giorda et al. [9] reported the results of a phase II trial in 42 patients that underwent surgery (radical hysterectomy) after 6–8 weeks of simultaneous chemotherapy and pelvic irradiation (50.4 Gy, 1.8 Gy/fraction). After the pathological study, only 5/35 (23%) of the patients achieved a complete response and gross macroscopical disease was present in 10/35 (26%) patients. After tumor removal, IORT was administered in 83% of the patients to parametria (82%), pelvic sidewalls, obturator fossa, iliac vessels, macroscopic residual tumor or macroscopic lymph nodes. IORT median given dose was 11 Gy (range between 10 and 15 Gy), being the median field size diameter 6.3 cm (range from 5.7 to 8.3 cm). At 5 years, the overall survival (OS) was 49% and the disease-free survival (DFS) was 46% with a median time to recurrence of 22 months. In this phase II trial, it was difficult to correlate the detected complications to IORT. Although the authors concluded that IORT was mainly effective in patients with a pathological complete response and in those with residual tumor limited to the cervix, this statement became very difficult to be demonstrated.

In a report from Foley et al. [10], 32 patients were treated with IORT after surgery over a period of 17 years (1994–2011) and 21 (65.6%) of them had a diagnosis of cervical cancer (locally advanced and recurrent cervical cancer). After surgery, 84.4% of the primary cervical cancer patients had microscopically positive margins. Patients were treated using electrons from IORT with a median dose of 13.5 Gy (range 10–22.5 Gy). The higher doses were delivered in the patients with gross tumor persistence. The mean cone size was 6.6 cm with diameters ranging between 4 and 10 cm. The pelvic sidewall was treated in 59.4%, central pelvis in 21.8% and para-aortic areas in 18.8%, respectively. Only one patient developed a grade 3 peripheral neuropathy and no other relevant complications were reported. The authors concluded on the usefulness of IORT after surgery in advanced cases and relapses from cervical cancer and remark the need for clinical trials to better analyze the benefit to add IORT to the surgery.

Gao et al. [11] reported the results of a series of 27 cases presenting a stage II cervical adenocarcinoma collected between 1999 and 2002. The rationale of the study was on the worse prognosis of this raising histological subtype. The patients underwent HDR (high dose rate) brachytherapy (overall dose of 12–14 Gy in 2 applications) and followed 1–2 weeks thereafter by surgery (total hysterectomy and selective lymphadenectomy). IORT given dose was 18–20 Gy using 12 MeV electrons and the diameter of the treatment field size was 10–12 cm with the protection of bowels, sigma, rectum and bladder. The obturator nerve was also partially shielded. Positive or close surgical margins were found in 8 of 27 cases (29.6%). About 4–6 courses of cisplatin and 5-fluorouracil adjuvant chemotherapy were administered 2 weeks after the surgery. The 5-year overall survival and disease-free survival were 77.8 and 70.4%, respectively. With a mean follow-up of 81 months, 2 patients developed local relapse (7.4%), but outside of the treatment field. The main complication was the peripheral neuropathy that appeared in 2 patients (7.4%) at 8 and 17 months, respectively. The authors concluded that IORT was safe and feasible, achieving an optimal local control benefit in stage II patients. The same group published in 2002 [12] a previous study describing the results of delivering IORT as a boosting irradiation technique after tumor resection in stage IIB patients. The 5-year survival was 95% and they conclude that this approach is a new and effective therapy method for this stage, mainly in adenocarcinoma histology.

According to the authors' conclusions, it is very difficult or perhaps near impossible to asses if adding IORT to extensive surgery in cervical cancer stage II has any advantage. Improving the results of standard therapies is not easy because the high control rates obtained. Even with a randomized trial, a large number of cases would be mandatory to have good discrimination and to be sure of a real benefit. We do not think that a study like that will be planned in a short future.

4. IORT in recurrent cervical cancer

Most of the IORT treatments in gynecological tumors have been performed in cervical cancer recurrences. The main locations of them are central pelvis (cervix or vaginal vault if previous radical hysterectomy), pelvic walls, parametria and nodal areas (pelvic or para-aortic). The IORT has been performed on the surgical bed after complete resection or over the remaining unresectable recurrence, mainly because of infiltration or adherence to vascular or other anatomical structures. Facing the optimal efficacy, the goal always will be to achieve a complete resection with surgical margin free (R0) or at least only microscopically invaded (R1). Clinical results became worse if residual gross tumor remains after surgery.

When we made a short review of published clinical data on IORT in cervical cancer recurrences, we found that all studies are retrospectives series. The recruitment periods are very long, with a low year rate and large heterogeneity in doses, irradiation fields, energies and duration of follow-up.

One of the historical series was published in 1997 by Garton et al. [13] from the Mayo Clinic. In a large group of 449 patients treated with IORT, 39 patients had gynecological tumors and 22 were cervical relapses. The median dose administered was 17.5 Gy (range 10– 25 Gy) and its variation was due to the different degrees of surgical radicality and tumor persistence (R0, R1 or R2). Most of the irradiated locations were lymph nodes followed by the pelvic wall. In a few cases, both sites were treated simultaneously. The 5-year actuarial local control rate on the irradiated area was 81% but decreased to 67% if the whole pelvic and nodal areas were registered. The 5-year DFS was 40.5% mainly due to the appearance of distant metastasis. The authors concluded that the association of surgery, IORT and, if possible, external beam radiotherapy was the right therapeutic approach, but with an uncertain benefit of including IORT.

One of the largest trials on recurrent cervical cancer is the study by Mahe et al. [14]. Due to the short survival registered in these patients, they made a retrospective revision of IORT-treated cases. Between 1985 and 1993, a cohort of 70 patients presenting with pelvic recurrences underwent IORT with or without external radiotherapy. The clinical series were collected from seven French institutions and results were reported in 1996. In most of the patients, the relapse location was on the pelvic sidewall (59/70) and central pelvis in the remaining patients. Lymph node relapses were not reported. Five patients underwent 100 kV X-rays IORT and electrons were used in the rest of the group. The median energy was 12 MeV (range 6–20 MeV) in R0/R1 cases and somewhat higher, 14 MeV (range 7–24 MeV), when macroscopic tumor persisted after surgery. The median IORT doses were similar (18–19 Gy) in both subgroups (R0/R1 vs. R2) but the broad range (10–30 Gy). The cone median diameter was 7.5 cm (range 4–9 cm). The median follow-up was 15 months and the 5-year actuarial local control was 21%, with an OS of only 8%. This study reported one of the lowest local control and survival rates in the literature. Five of seventy patients (7.1%) developed late peripheral neuropathy, presenting with pain and paresthesia. The authors concluded that IORT seems feasible in recurrent cervical cancer but cannot dramatically improve prognosis.

A second paper from the Mayo Clinic was published some years later, in 2013, by Barney et al. [15]. The recruiting period was extended 9 years, with a total of 86 patients treated between 1983 and 2010. Eight-five percent of patients had locally recurrent tumors and the remaining patients locally advanced primary cervical cancer. The most commonly performed surgery associated with IORT was pelvic exenteration (30%) followed by pelvic side wall resection (26%). In 20% of the patients, IORT was delivered to metastatic para-aortic nodes. During the surgical procedure, 67% of the cases were found involving the pelvic sidewall but maximal debulking surgery was performed. Surgical margins were free (R0) in 41% of cases, microscopically involved (R1) in 35% and gross residual tumor (R2) in 24%. The patients underwent IORT with an electron beam from a conventional linear accelerator. The median given dose was 15 Gy (range 6–25 Gy) according to the resection margin (R0, R1 or R2). Site and R status were the parameters used to select the appropriate beam energies, and 9 and 12 MeV were the most commonly employed. In the previous study from the same institution [13], the median dose was a little higher (17.5 Gy vs. 15 Gy) and the irradiated volume slightly smaller in the present series. The authors considered that combining IORT and pelvic exenteration, the best results were achieved, improving the probability of local control. After surgery, an R0 or R1 pathological result was obtained only in half of the patients, but the 3-year actuarial local control was 56%. Also, only 43% of patients underwent external beam irradiation after surgery. About IORT-related toxicity, 16/89 (18%) patients experienced peripheral neuropathy, 4/89 (4.5%) ureteral stenosis and also 4.5% bowel perforation or fistula. We must point out that, keeping in mind that both studies from the Mayo Clinic share most of the patients, local control rates are rather different (70% at 5 years vs. 56% at 3 years). The authors concluded that long-term survival is possible with combined modality therapy including IORT for advanced and recurrences of cervical cancer, but distant relapse is common.

A Spanish study by Sole et al. [16] published in 2014 evaluated a series of 31 patients with recurrent cervical cancer. Because all patients had undergone previous external irradiation, the management of relapse was limited to complete or debulking surgical resection and IORT. The mean electron given dose was 12.5 Gy (range 10 to 15 Gy) and the median beam energy 12 Mev from a standard linear accelerator. Circular cones most beveled ranged from 5 to 12 cm in diameter. The 5-year actuarial local control, OS and DFS were 65, 42, and 44%, respectively. Secondary effects directly associated with IORT were not reported. The authors concluded that patients presenting with local or nodal relapse were safely treated and had improved local control by adding IORT to the surgical resection. The largest benefit was detected in the R0 cases.

Tran et al. [17] conducted a study at Stanford University and reported the clinical results of a retrospective series of 36 consecutive patients treated from 1986 to 2005. Cervical recurrent tumors were present in 17 (47%) patients, and all of them had negative margins (R0) on the perioperative pathological examination. IORT was delivered with an orthovoltage X-ray equipment (200–250 kV), using circular cones with diameters from 2.5 to 10 cm and bevels between 0° and 45°. Doses were referred to as the surface of the surgical bed. In some patients, customized lead shielding was designed to protect neighboring radiosensitive organs. The median dose given was 11.5 Gy (range 6–17.5 Gy). The 5-year actuarial local control was 45% and the DSF 46%. These results, which were more favorable than those reported elsewhere, should be interpreted taking into account that IORT was only administered in patients with R0 resections. Another explanation was the lower rate of sidewall pelvic location, 32% vs. 84% in the French study [16]. As previously commented on, recurrences on the pelvic sidewall have the worst prognosis compared with other sites such as the central pelvis or isolated metastatic lymph nodes. A very low reported rate of secondary effects due to IORT may be explained by shielding the organs at risk and limiting the peripheral nerve dose below 12.5 Gy. As a conclusion and remarking the importance of wisely selecting the candidates to IORT, the authors colloquially wrote: "It is a question of fishing in the right hole".

A few years ago, in 2014, Backes et al. [18] published an article investigating whether the association of pelvic exenteration and IORT in recurrent gynecological cancer could improve survival. A total of 21 patients out of 32 (65.6%) with recurrence of cervical cancer underwent surgical resection and IORT. The median radiation dose was 17.5 Gy (range 10–20 Gy). The selected electron beam energy ranged from 6 to 12 MeV and the dose depth prescription was, as usual, at 90% isodose curve. In eight patients, the intraoperative radiation was delivered with HDR brachytherapy catheters. It is difficult to understand the results given only 66% (21/32) of patients received IORT and the origin of the primary tumor (cervix, endometrium) was unclear. Probably the reason for that may be explained because the review has been focused to evaluate the efficacy of pelvic exenteration in the whole series. The 5-year actuarial local control rate differs according to the extension of surgery: pelvic exenteration and IORT (64%) vs. laterally extended endopelvic resection (69%). The authors' conclusions remarked that IORT fails to ameliorate local control and survival outcomes. Nevertheless, the cohort treated with pelvic exenteration and IORT had a worse prognosis compared with patients treated only with pelvis lateral wall surgery. It would reasonable to conclude that if the local control rates are similar in both arms the addition of IORT may contribute to raising the local control in the worst prognosis subgroup.

To our knowledge, the most recent reported study on gynecological malignancies treated with surgery and IORT is the German study of Arians et al. [19] published in 2016. This retrospective series included 36 patients, 18 (50%) of whom presented with cervical cancer recurrence. The recruitment period was 12 years (2002–2014). IORT was performed with a mobile linear accelerator delivering a range of electron beam energies between 6 and 18 MeV. Radiosensitive organs (bowel, ureters and peripheral nerves) were displaced out of the irradiated field or using radiation protection lead shields. The median given dose was 15 Gy (range 10–18 Gy) and the median energy 8 MeV (range 6–15 MeV). The maximum dose permitted to the nerves was always below 10–12 Gy. With a median follow-up of 14 months, the actuarial 5-year OS rate was 6.4% and the DFS 0%. The results of local control were even worse, with a rate of 0% at 2 years. The reported neural toxicity was 11%. Based on these unfavorable results, the authors concluded that surgical resection and IORT in cervical cancer recurrence should be considered a rather palliative procedure, suggesting a careful selection of patients to identify those who may benefit from this combined approach.

Our institutional experience is still limited and has been partially reported [20]. The IORT program started in 2013 with a mobile electron linear accelerator (LIAC) installed in a specifically designed operation room. Treatment objectives are mainly focused on conservative breast cancer but a series of patients with gynecological cancer recurrence have also been included as candidates to receive IORT. At present, 16 patients have been enrolled. Primary tumors included uterine cervix in 11 patients, uterine corpus in 4 and ovarian cancer in 1. The mean age was 53 years (range 40–68). The most common histological type has been squamous cell carcinoma (10/16) followed by different types of adenocarcinoma (5/16) and one carcinosarcoma. Hysterectomy was performed in six cases, resection of local recurrence lesions in five and pelvic exenteration in five. A negative pathological margin (R0) was obtained in 9/16 cases, microscopically involved margins (R1) in 6/16 and macroscopic residual tumor in 1. IORT was administered to the surgical bed using an electron beam with energy ranges from 4 to 12 MeV and a mean diameter field of 5 cm (range 4–6). The median prescribed dose has been 11 Gy (range 8–15 Gy). We consider that beyond 15 Gy the probability of peripheral nerve damage is not acceptable. All the irradiated patients presented with pelvic recurrences (central in eight, the pelvic wall in four and both sites in four) but the involvement of para-aortic nodes was also present in two patients. At follow-up, there were five cancer deaths and two patients were lost. Eight patients are in complete remission without any recurrence in the irradiated area. Only one marginal relapse has appeared.

Taken all these data together, the difficulties of obtaining valid and objective conclusions should be emphasized. The heterogeneity of the data, size, location, and extent of the relapses, the different therapeutic approaches, IORT doses, different surgical procedures, etc. must be taken into account before inadequate conclusions. Probably, adding IORT to the debulking surgery may give an extra benefit in terms of local control, particularly if the resection is R0 or R1. But the influence on survival seems, if any, poor because of the high probability to develop pelvic carcinomatosis or distant metastasis.

5. Endometrial cancer

The experience with IORT in endometrial cancer is still more limited than in cervical cancer. Firstly, the pattern of recurrence is different, with very infrequent isolated relapses in the vaginal fundus fulfilling surgical indication. Most are usually controlled by external radiotherapy and brachytherapy. In other cases, the recurrence is in the form of peritoneal carcinomatosis, which already rules out combined management of surgery and IORT.

When reviewing the literature, it is observed that the majority of revisions do not include cases of endometrial cancer or do not allow their identification because they are mixed with the most numerous of the cervix or even vagina and vulva. For example, Solé et al. [16] in a series of 62 cases recruited over 17 years acknowledge that they have not included the origin of the primary tumor in the analysis criteria. In a subsequent article published 1 year later (2015) [21] dedicated specifically to IORT in oligometastases of gynecological cancer, it is surprising that it refers to more cases of endometrial than of cervical origin (18 vs. 14). With an average follow-up of 55 months, local control was 79% and DFS 44%, which stimulates the addition of IORT to external radiotherapy. In the multivariate analysis, surgery with a positive margin (R1) was the only independent prognostic factor. In a historical series of the Mayo Clinic, published in 1997 by Garton et al. [22] that includes 39 gynecological neoplasms (recurrent or advanced), only 7 are primary endometrial tumors.

In the aforementioned review carried out by Backes et al. [4], 276 cases of cervical cancer with IORT from 8 institutions were collected, but there were only 52 cases of endometrial cancer. This can be explained by the encouraging results of the primary treatment and even of the few isolated vaginal recurrences registered, which through a combination of external radiotherapy and brachytherapy reached control rates between 60% and 70%. Dowdy et al. [23] described a series of 25 patients with recurrence of endometrial cancer treated by external radiotherapy, surgical resection and IORT. The probability of local control was 84% but dropped to 47% if residual tumor persisted. For this reason, they insisted on the need to achieve surgery with negative margins. The two cases with isolated para-aortic relapses achieved control of the disease. Awtrey et al. [24] in 2006, 26 months after that study of Dowdy et al. [23], published a second specific study of IORT and endometrial cancer.

One of the main difficulties to get any valid conclusion about the usefulness of IORT is the great disparity between different studies. Nowadays, endometrial cancer has a good prognosis in most of the treated cases. Recurrences are scarce and 80% of them are located in the vaginal vault. Standard treatment of brachytherapy with or without external radiotherapy obtains satisfactory results. The cases that underwent surgery may benefit from the addition of IORT. The IORT published results in endometrium-isolated relapses are better than in cervical cancer and the toxicity is assumable if doses are under 15 Gy. We must keep in mind that a significant number of patients will present later on peritoneal carcinomatosis and/ or lung metastasis, mainly the grade III tumors. Finally, it is slightly surprising that, in the cases presenting bad prognostic factors, IORT is not used more, because local control in endometrial cancer is mandatory.

6. Ovarian cancer

In most published studies, the cases of IORT in ovarian cancer are marginal and scarce, so that it is difficult to achieve any conclusions. As far as we are aware, there are only four relevant studies on the role of IORT in ovarian cancer.

One of the oldest series is that of Konski et al. [25] in 1990. They performed IORT on nine patients with recurrence of ovarian cancer and compared their evolution with a similar group without IORT. Survival was similar in both groups.

Yap et al. [26] present a series of 24 patients undergoing cytoreductive surgery with which IORT was delivered to the areas at high risk of residual disease. Interestingly, IORT was given by using a 200 kV X-ray beam instead of an electron beam. The average dose was 12 Gy (range 9–14 Gy). At 2 years follow-up, only 5 of the 24 patients were in complete remission, but only 5 showed relapse in the irradiated surgical bed, and the remaining relapse occurred in other areas. Because of the results, they concluded that IORT had some activity but its influence on the prognosis was very limited.

A more extensive series is the experience of Gao et al. [27] with 45 patients enrolled along 11 years (2000–2010) and undergoing cytoreductive surgery. IORT was performed on the pelvis using larger than usual fields (10–12 cm in diameter) and higher than usual doses, 18–20 Gy except in two cases with 10 Gy. They register local faults by 32% but the majority outside the irradiated field (10/14). The DFS was 55% at 5 years. The authors reported a rate of peripheral neuropathy of 11%, with an average time elapsed period of 11 months (range 8–22). They also register 4% of hydronephrosis. It was concluded that IORT was effective in advanced cases or recurrences undergoing surgery, as well as it appears to discreetly increase survival and quality of life. Toxicity attributable to given doses greater than 15 Gy was not mentioned.

Barney et al. [28] from the Mayo Clinic published in 2011 a series of 20 cases treated between 1987 and 2009 because of relapses after surgery and chemotherapy. The IORT zones were pelvis (14/20), para-aortic (6/20) and inguinal fields. The average electron dose was 12.5 Gy (range 10–22.5 Gy). The probability of global-local control at 5 years was 59%, with 76% in the irradiated volume. In all cases of recurrence in the irradiation field, surgeries were R1. Survival at 5 years was 49%, similar to that in the previous study. Neural toxicity was recorded in three cases (15%).

Finally, Albuquerque et al. [29] reported a series of 27 localized extraperitoneal recurrences of ovarian cancer. In 17 cases (63%), surgical results R0 or R1 were obtained. At 5 years, the probability of local control in the irradiated area was 70% and DFS was 33%. It should be noted that in this series 37% of patients had macroscopic disease after surgery. The authors make a comparison with a similar group of relapsed patients treated only with surgery and chemotherapy without finding significant differences in survival, but they concluded "suggesting a role for locoregional therapies in selected patients presenting recurrences in ovarian cancer."

The role and possible benefit of adding IORT to the surgical resection in ovarian cancers' localized recurrences are still under debate. These kinds of recurrences, tumoral or nodal, are infrequent. Survival is not modified and probably the local control is more related to the quality of life. As we consider ovarian cancer as more a systemic disease and focus more on systemic therapy, we can assess than IORT would have only a role in the scarce cases presenting an isolated and resectable pelvic recurrence.

7. Miscellaneous

In this section, we would like to comment briefly on three publications as a whole, in which no distinction has been made according to the origin of the gynecological neoplasia. The first one, from Coelho et al. [30], retrospectively analyzed 41 patients with isolated or retroperitoneal recurrences of colorectal, gynecological or retroperitoneal primary tumors. Following salvage surgery, all patients underwent tumor bed IORT with an electron beam or brachytherapy. The median dose of IORT was 12 Gy. A total of 15 gynecological cancers (36%) were included, including tumors of the cervix in 8 cases, uterine corpus in 6 and ovary in 1. Patients were enrolled along 11 years, between 2004 and 2015, with a rate of 1.3 cases per year. The 5-year local control rate was 81%. Surgery R1 was the worst prognostic factor. Peripheral neural toxicity occurred in 7% of the cases.

Haddock et al. [31] reported the results of a retrospective series of 63 patients treated during a period of 12 years (1983–1995). The recruiting rate was 5.25 cases/year. IORT was administered in 8 primary gynecological tumors and 55 relapses. Most of the patients (n = 40) had cervical cancer. There were 16 patients with tumors of the endometrium, 5 with vaginal and 2 with ovarian. Most patients had been previously treated with external beam radiotherapy. IORT was given with electrons with a range of energies between 9 and 18 MeV. When macroscopic residual persisted after surgery, the median dose administered was 20 Gy (R2) and 15 Gy in R0-R1 cases. The actuarial 5-year local control was 74% but the probability to survive was 27%. The authors concluded that long-term disease control is obtainable in a significant number of carefully selected patients with locally advanced or recurrent gynecological malignancies with aggressive multimodality treatment, including IORT. Disease control was better when gross total resection was possible. Patients with local or regional relapse after previous external beam radiotherapy appeared to fare as well as those previously non-irradiated.

Finally, Gemignani et al. [32] reported a short series of 17 patients diagnosed with gynecological tumor recurrences. They were treated over a period of 5 years (1993–1998) with an inclusion rate of 3.4 cases per year, quite similar to our recruiting rate. Surprisingly, they are very young, with a median age of only 49 years (range 27 to 72). The origin of neoplasms was the cervix in nine patients, the endometrium in seven and the vagina in one. R0-R1 surgical resections were obtained in 76% of cases and the median IORT dose was 14 Gy. The actuarial 3-year local control reached 67% but if gross tumor remains after surgery the local control decreased to 25%. In R0-R1 cases, the actuarial 3-year control was the highest, with an 85% rate, but the DFS rate was 54%. Peripheral neuropathy occurred in 18% of cases and ureteral stenosis in 12%. The authors concluded the need to obtain R0-R1 surgical resections.

The results of different series obtained in clinical practice with the use of IORT in patients with gynecological cancer are shown in **Table 1**. Most of the experience comes from resected recurrences in various locations, mainly in the central pelvis. Cervical cancer is the most frequent diagnosis followed by endometrium and ovary. The most relevant published experience since 1995 includes 727 patients. The median number of patients per institution is 36, taking into account that the 70 cases described by the French collaborative study [16] came from 7 institutions. The median given dose has been 14.8 Gy but with large differences (range between 27

YEAR	Reference	N	Classification	IORT median dose and range in Grays	5y OS	5y DFS	5y LC
1995	Stelzer et al. [33]	22	Recurrent	22 (14–27)	43%	—	48%
1996	Mahe et al. [14]	70	Recurrent	18 (10–25)	8%(3y)	—	30%
1997	Haddock et al. [31]	63	Mix	15 (8–25)	26%	—	67%
1997	Garton et al. [13]	39	Mix	17 (10–25)	40%	32%	76%
2001	Martinez-Monge et al. [8]	36	Recurrent	15	14%	16%	42%
2001	Martinez-Monge et al. [8]	31	Primary-cervix	12	67%	70%	79%
2001	Gemignani et al. [32]	17	Recurrent	14 (12–15)	54% 3y	54% 3y	83% 3y
2002	Liu and Chen [12]	97	Primary-cervix	19 (18–20)	88%	—	—
2005	Yap et al. [26]	24	Recurrent-ovary	12 (9–14)	22%	—	68%
2006	Dowdy et al. [23]	25	Recurrent	15 (10–25)	71%	—	—
2007	Tran et al. [17]	36	Recurrent	11 (6–17)	—	47%	44%
2011	Giorda et al. [9]	35	Primary-cervix	11 (10–15)	49%	46%	89%
2013	Gao et al. [27]	27	Primary-cervix	19 (18–20)	78%	70%	100%
2013	Barney et al. [15]	73	Recurrent	15 (6–25)	—	31%	61%
2013	Barney et al. [15]	13	Primary-cervix	15 (6–25)	—	—	70%
2014	Foley et al. [10]	21	Recurrent	13.5 (10–22)	69%	30%	59%
2014	Backes and Martin [4]	21	Recurrent	17.5 (10–20)	30%	—	59%
2015	Sole et al. [21]	61	Recurrent	12 (10–15)	42%	44%	65%
2016	Arians et al. [19]	36	Recurrent	15 (10–18)	22%	—	44%
2018	Biete and Oses [20]	16	Recurrent	11 (8–15)	79%	—	86%
2018	Coelho et al. [30]	15	Recurrent	12 (9–15)	56%	—	81%

OS, overall survival; DFS, disease-free survival; LC, local control.

Table 1.
Selected studies of the use of IORT for gynecologic malignancies.

and 6 Gy). We have divided all groups into two periods: 1995–2007 and 2008–2018. The median dose in the first period has been 15.5 Gy (range 6–27 Gy), whereas the median dose in the second period was 14.1 Gy (range 6–25 Gy). Differences are minor but a tendency to slightly lower doses is detected. The higher doses were administered when gross residual tumor persisted after surgery (R2) assuming that doses over 15 Gy increase the risk of peripheral neural toxicity and may cause ureteral stenosis and pelvic fibrosis if these structures are irradiated. However, in daily clinical practice, it is difficult to determine the precise cause of secondary effects: surgery, radiation or both. Broad differences in local control results are also registered. The probability to be free of the treated recurrence at 5 years switched around 30 and 100%, but most percentages are about 70–80%. No comparisons are allowed due to the high degree of heterogeneity among studies. **Table 2** shows the

Author	Period	Years	N	Rate/year
Coelho et al. [30]	2004–2005	11	15	1.4
Foley et al. [10]	1994–2011	17	32	1.9
Sole et al. [16]	1997–2012	15	35	2.3
Garton et al. [13]	1983–1991	8	39	4.9
Backes and Martin [4]	2000–2012	13	21	1.6
Arians et al. [19]	2002–2014	12	36	3.0
Tran et al. [17]	1986–2005	20	36	1.8
Giorda et al. [9]	2000–2007	8	42	5.2
Gao et al. [11]	1999–2006	7	27	3.8
Barney et al. [15]	1983–2010	27	86	3.2
Mahe et al. [14]	1985–1993	8	70	8.7
Gemignani et al. [32]	1993–1998	6	17	2.8
Garton et al. [22]	1981–1992	11	42	3.8
Martinez-Monge et al. [8]	1985–1992	8	26	3.2
Haddock et al. [31]	1983–1995	13	63	4.8
Dowdy et al. [23]	1986–2002	16	25	1.6
Yap et al. [26]	1994–2002	9	24	2.7
Biete and Oses [20]	2013–2017	5	16	3.2

Table 2.
Recruitment period and year rate of different authors' published studies.

different recruiting rates from 18 studies, with a median study period of 10.7 years, although there is a large variation between a minimum of 5 years and a maximum of 27 years. The total number of cases included in this table is 626 and the median of cases per institution is 34.7 (range 15–86). The median recruitment rate is low (3.2 cases/year) and ranges between a maximum of 5.2 cases/year and a minimum of 1.4 cases/year. The previously cited French study raises a rate of 8.7 cases/year, but if we consider the 7 different institutions, then the rate lowers to 1.2 cases/year per hospital. Recruitment rates have been stable over the years, and also a strong heterogeneity in the published series persists.

8. Conclusions

The published studies on IORT have many parameters of heterogeneity. Some of them are as follows: recurrence sites of different prognosis such as pelvic sidewalls or central pelvic, margin status on resection (R0, R1 or R2), tumor initial and residual burden, high level of heterogeneity according to the different techniques, energies, fields, doses, etc. Even more, the conclusions of the referred studies are frequently different. It is not easy to demonstrate the efficacy and the benefit of IORT in these retrospective limited series. IORT is a radiation boost in a surgical procedure. In well-designed randomized prospective studies, it is frequently difficult to demonstrate the degree of local control benefit of postoperative radiotherapy. This is particularly difficult in IORT because it is necessarily associated with different degrees of radicality in surgery, from local resection to pelvic exenteration or simply debulking.

However, most of the referred studies agree that adding IORT to surgical resection is the right strategy for raising the local control rate. There are more doubts about the influence on survival and probably there is a little impact. Nevertheless, in cervical cancer, local control has a strong impact on the quality of life. We must keep in mind that half of the mortality in cervical cancer is due to a non-controlled pelvic disease.

By contrast, the therapeutic approach in primary tumors, including surgery and IORT, is strongly debated. It seems there is no clear advantage over the standard well-established approach, including chemoradiotherapy and brachytherapy. But there is some agreement that, if surgery is the therapeutic option, IORT is an effective tool adding extra safety and increasing the local control rate. Nevertheless, IORT is a therapeutical option still not included in the clinical guides.

Finally, we must point out the difficulty and the low probability to design and conduct randomized prospective trials. The experienced low accrual of enough number of patients in a reasonable time and the heterogeneity of recurrences and surgical procedures are hard difficulties to overcome.

9. Concluding remarks

Most of the published studies on IORT on gynecological cancer collected small and non-homogeneous series of patients with the additional difficulty of the long enrolment period. Cervical cancer, as primary or recurrence, is the most analyzed tumor, but many studies include a blend of recurrences from different sites: endometrium, ovary and vagina. At the same time, there is a broad variety of recurrence locations: central pelvis, pelvic walls, retroperitoneal or pelvic nodes are the most common. There is also a great variation of the surgical radicality and margin status: R0, R1 or R2.

Nowadays, knowledge comes from retrospective and heterogeneous series. High survival achieved on the primary treatment, mainly in the cervix and endometrium, results in the onset of a few local recurrences. Then, candidates for IORT are scarce and the recruitment rate becomes low in all the institutions. On the other hand, IORT is not a standard option at the initial treatment. Even taken into account all the difficulties explained before, there is a broad consensus that IORT as a radiation boost after salvage surgery adds an extra benefit to achieve better local control. Also, some authors assess that survival may also be slightly increased. There is no doubt about the benefit of IORT on quality of life. Even in patients presenting with the metastatic disease, local control is a valuable goal and has a substantial impact on the quality of life.

An important challenge for the future is the control of the tumor spreading in the peritoneal cavity, and in this case, the impact of the recurrence local control utilizing surgery and IORT would raise. Probably there will be in the near future little changes in IORT technique delivery excepting smaller units with better mobility and versatility. A significant increase in the treated patients' rate is not expected, quite different from conservative breast cancer treatment.

Finally, the limited side effects of this radiation modality if doses do not exceed 15 Gy must stick out. However, after nearly 30 years, IORT remains a technique of uneasy availability due to the limited number of institutions where it is available.

DOI: http://dx.doi.org/10.5772/intechopen.91641

Author details

Albert Biete[1*], Angeles Rovirosa[1] and Gabriela Oses[2]

1 Radiation Oncology Department and Gynecological Oncology Unit, Hospital Clinic, University of Barcelona, Spain

2 Radiation Oncology Department and Breast Unit, Hospital Clinic, University of Barcelona, Spain

*Address all correspondence to: abiete@ub.edu

References

[1] Beck C. On external roentgen treatment of internal structures. New York Medical Journal. 1909;**89**: 621-622

[2] Casas F, Ferrer C, Calvo FA. European historical note of intraoperative radiation therapy (IORT). A case report from 1905. Radiotherapy and Oncology. 1997;**43**:323-324

[3] Comas C, Prio A. Irradiation roentgen preventive intra-abdominal, après l'intervention chirurgicale dans un cas de cancer de l'uterus: Communication au III Congrés International d'Electro-radiologie. Barcelona: Francisco Badia; 1906. p. 1907

[4] Backes F, Martin D. Intraoperative radiation therapy (IORT) for gynecologic malignancies. Gynecologic Oncology. 2015;**138**:449-456

[5] Krengli M, Pisani C, Deantonio L, Surico D, et al. Intraoperative radiotherapy for gynecological and genitourinary malignancies: Focus on endometrial, cervical, renal, bladder and prostate cancers. Radiation Oncology. 2017;**12**:18-27

[6] Belletti B, Vaidya S, D'Andrea S, Entschladen F, et al. Targeted intraoperative radiotherapy impairs the stimulation of breast cancer cell proliferation and invasion caused by surgical wounding. Clinical Cancer Research. 2008;**14**:1325-1331

[7] Zaleska K, Suchorska WM, Przybyla A, Murawa D. Effect of surgical wound fluids after intraoperative electron radiotherapy on the cancer stem cell phenotype in a panel of human breast cancer cell lines. Oncology Letters. 2016;**12**:3707-3714

[8] Martinez-Monge R, Jurado M, Aristu JJ, Moreno M, et al. Intraoperative electron beam radiotherapy during radical surgery for locally advanced and recurrent cervical cancer. Gynecologic Oncology. 2001;**82**:538-543

[9] Giorda G, Boz G, Gadducci A, Lucia E, et al. Multimodality approach in extra-cervical locally advanced cervical cancer: Chemoradiation, surgery and intra-operative radiation therapy. A phase II trial. EJSO. 2011;**37**:442-447

[10] Foley O, Rauh-Hain JA, Clark R, Goodman A, et al. Intraoperative radiation therapy in the management of gynecologic malignancies. American Journal of Clinical Oncology. 2016;**39**:329-334

[11] Gao Y, Liu Z, Gao F, Chen X. Intraoperative radiotherapy in stage IIB adenocarcinoma of the uterine cervix: A retrospective study. Oncotargets and Therapy. 2013;**6**:1695-1700

[12] Liu Z, Chen X. Preliminary results of intraoperative radiation therapy for cervical carcinoma IIB. Zhonghua Fu Chan Ke Za Zhi. 2002;**37**:553-555

[13] Garton GR, Gunderson L, Webb M, Wilson T, et al. Intraoperative radiation therapy in gynecologic cancer: The Mayo Clinic experience. Gynecologic Oncology. 1993;**48**:328-332

[14] Mahe MA, Gerard JP, Dubois JB, Roussel A, et al. Intraoperative radiation therapy in recurrent carcinoma of the uterine cervix: Report of the French intraoperative group on 70 patients. International Journal of Radiation Oncology, Biology, Physics. 1996;**34**:21-26

[15] Barney B, Petersen I, Dowdy S, Bakkum-Gamez N, et al. Intraoperative electron beam radiotherapy (IOERT) in the management of locally advanced or recurrent cervical cancer. Radiation Oncology. 2013;**8**:80-89

[16] Sole CV, Calvo FA, Lozano MA, Gonzalez-Bayon L, et al. External-beam radiation therapy after surgical resection and intraoperative electron beam radiation therapy for oligorecurrent gynecological cancer. Long-term outcome. Strahlentherapie und Onkologie. 2014;**190**:171-180

[17] Tran P, Su Z, Hara W, Husain M, et al. Long-term survivors using intraoperative radiotherapy for recurrent gynecological malignancies. International Journal of Radiation Oncology, Biology, Physics. 2007;**69**(2): 504-511

[18] Backes F, Billingsley C, Martin D, Tierney B, et al. Does intra-operative radiation at the time of pelvic exenteration improve survival for patients for recurrent previously irradiated cervical, vaginal or vulvar cancer? Gynecologic Oncology. 2014;**135**:95-99

[19] Arians N, Foerster R, Rom J, Uhl M, et al. Outcome of patients with local recurrent gynecological malignancies after resection combined with intraoperative electron radiation therapy (IOERT). Radiation Oncology. 2016;**11**:44-54

[20] Biete A, Oses G. Radiation therapy in uterine cervical cancer: A review. Reports of Practical Oncology and Radiotherapy. 2018;**23**:589-594

[21] Sole CV, Calvo FA, Lizarraga S, Gonzalez-Bayon L, Garcia-Sabrido JL. Intraoperative electron-beam radiation therapy with or without external beam radiotherapy in the management of paraaortic lymph-node oligometastases from gynecological malignancies. Clinical & Translational Oncology. 2015;**17**:910-916

[22] Garton GR, Gunderson LL, Webb MJ, Wilson TO, Cha SS, Podrazt KC. Intraoperative radiation therapy in gynecologic cancer: Update of the experience at a single institution. International Journal of Radiation Oncology, Biology, Physics. 1997;**37**:839-843

[23] Dowdy SC, Mariani A, Clibby VA, Haddock MG, Petersen IA, Sim FH, et al. Radical pelvic resection and intraoperative radiotherapy for recurrent endometrial cancer: Technique and analysis of outcomes. Gynecologic Oncology. 2006;**101**:280-286

[24] Awtrey C, Cadungog M, Leitao M, et al. Surgical resection for endometrial carcinoma. Gynecologic Oncology. 2006;**102**:480-488

[25] Konski A, Neisler J, Phibbs B, et al. A pilot study investigating intraoperative electron beam irradiation in the treatment of ovarian malignancies. Gynecologic Oncology. 1990;**38**:121-124

[26] Yap OW, Kapp DS, Teng NN, et al. Intraoperative radiation therapy in recurrent ovarian cancer. International Journal of Radiation Oncology, Biology, Physics. 2005;**63**:1114-1121

[27] Gao Y, Liu Z, Chen X, et al. Intraoperative radiotherapy electron boost in advanced and recurrent ovarian epithelial carcinoma: A retrospective study. BMC Cancer. 2011;**11**:439

[28] Barney BM, Petersen IA, Dowdy SC, et al. Intraoperative electron beam radiotherapy in the management of recurrent ovarian malignancies. International Journal of Gynecological Cancer. 2011;**21**:1225-1231

[29] Albuquerque K, Patel M, Liotta M, et al. Long-term benefit of tumor-volume directed involved field radiation therapy in the management of recurrent ovarian cancer. International Journal of Gynecological Cancer. 2016;**26**:4

[30] Coelho TM, Fogaroli RC, Pellizzon AC, et al. Intraoperative

radiation therapy for the treatment of recurrent retroperitoneal and pelvic tumors: A single-institution analysis. Radiation Oncology. 2018;**13**:224-237

[31] Haddock MG, Petersen IA, Webb MJ. IORT for locally advanced malignancies. Frontiers of Radiation Therapy and Oncology. 1997;**31**:256-259

[32] Gemignani ML, Alektiar KM, Leitao M, et al. Radical surgical resection and high dose intraoperative radiotherapy in patients with recurrent gynecologic cancers. International Journal of Radiation Oncology, Biology, Physics. 2001;**50**:687-694

[33] Stelzer KJ, Kohn WJ, Greer BE, et al. The use of intraoperative radiotherapy in radical salvage surgery for recurrent cervical cancer: Outcome and toxicity. American Journal of Obstetrics and Gynecology. 1995;**172**:1881-1886